ESSENTIAL

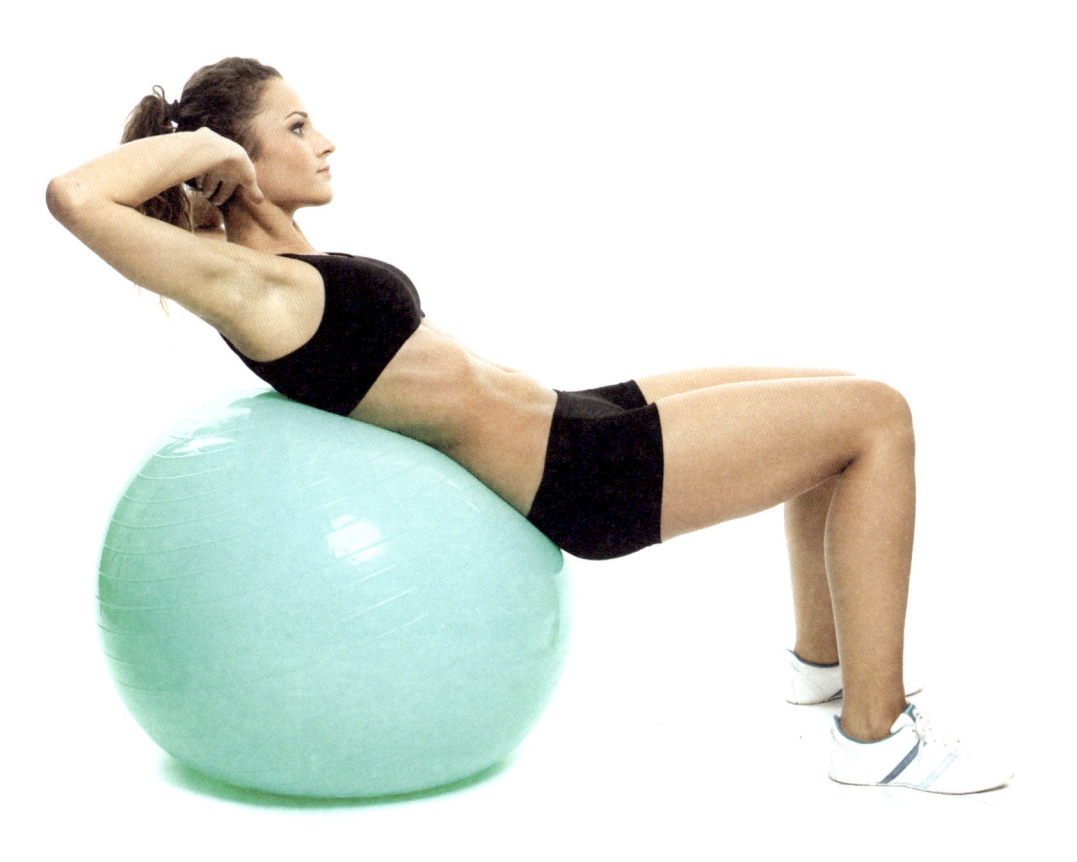

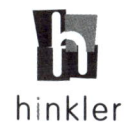

Ball

hinkler

Published by Hinkler Books Pty Ltd
45–55 Fairchild Street
Heatherton, VIC 3202, Australia
www.hinkler.com.au

hinkler

Text © Hinkler Books Pty Ltd 2003
Design © Hinkler Books Pty Ltd 2003, 2016

Prepress: Graphic Print Group
Authors: Jennifer Pohlman and Rodney Searle
Editor: Margaret Barca
Photography: Peter Wakeman
Cover design: Sam Grimmer

Images © Hinkler Books Pty Ltd or Shutterstock.com

All rights reserved. No part of this publication may be reproduced, stored in a retrieval system, or transmitted in any way or by any means, electronic, mechanical, photocopying, recording or otherwise, without the prior written permission of Hinkler Books Pty Ltd.

ISBN: 978 1 4889 2964 9

Printed and bound in China

When exercising on the ball, always do the warm up exercises before attempting any individual exercises. It is recommended that you check with your doctor or healthcare professional before commencing any exercise regime. Whilst every care has been taken in the preparation of this material, the publishers and their respective employees or agents will not accept responsibility for injury or damage occasioned to any person as a result of participation in the activities described in this book.

CONTENTS

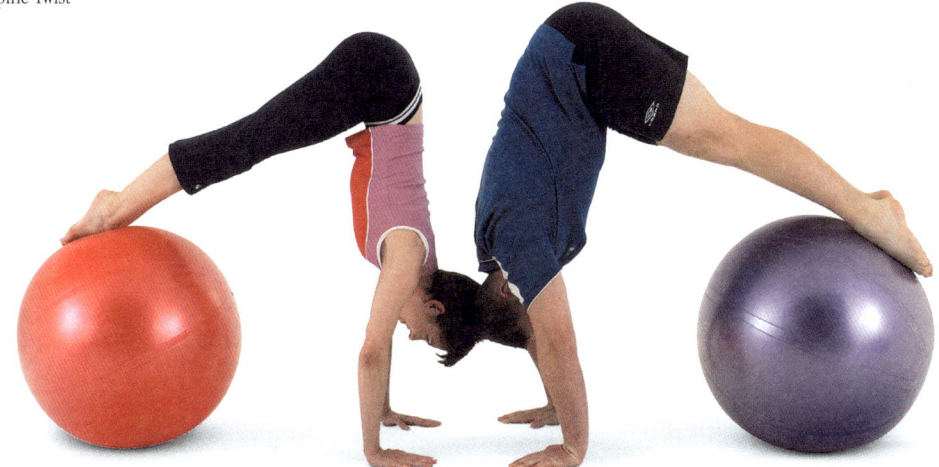

INTRODUCTION 5

THE BENEFITS 9

PRACTICAL MATTERS 10

CENTRING & BREATHING 12

BREATHING EXERCISE 14

POSTURE AWARENESS
& ABDOMINAL PREPARATION 16
Seated Balance, Pelvic Tilt, Chest Lift on the Ball

ABDOMINAL STRENGTHENING
& PELVIC STABILITY 22
Leg Pull, Chest Lift, Oblique Lifts, Roll Up Prep,
Double Leg Stretch, Single Leg Stretch

SPINAL MOBILITY & CONTROL 34
Side to Side, Pelvic Tilt, Rollover Prep, Rollovers

SPINAL ROTATION 42
Spine Twist

GLUTEALS & ADDUCTORS 44
Bottom Lift Series, Side Balance

SCAPULA STABILITY
& BACK STRENGTHENING 48
Arm Openings, Back Extension

FULL BODY INTEGRATION 52
Leg Beats, Push-ups

STRETCH & RELAX 56
Thoracic Push Through, Overhead Reach,
Hamstring Stretch, Hip Flexor Stretch

GLOSSARY 62

CONCLUSION 63

ABOUT THE AUTHORS 64

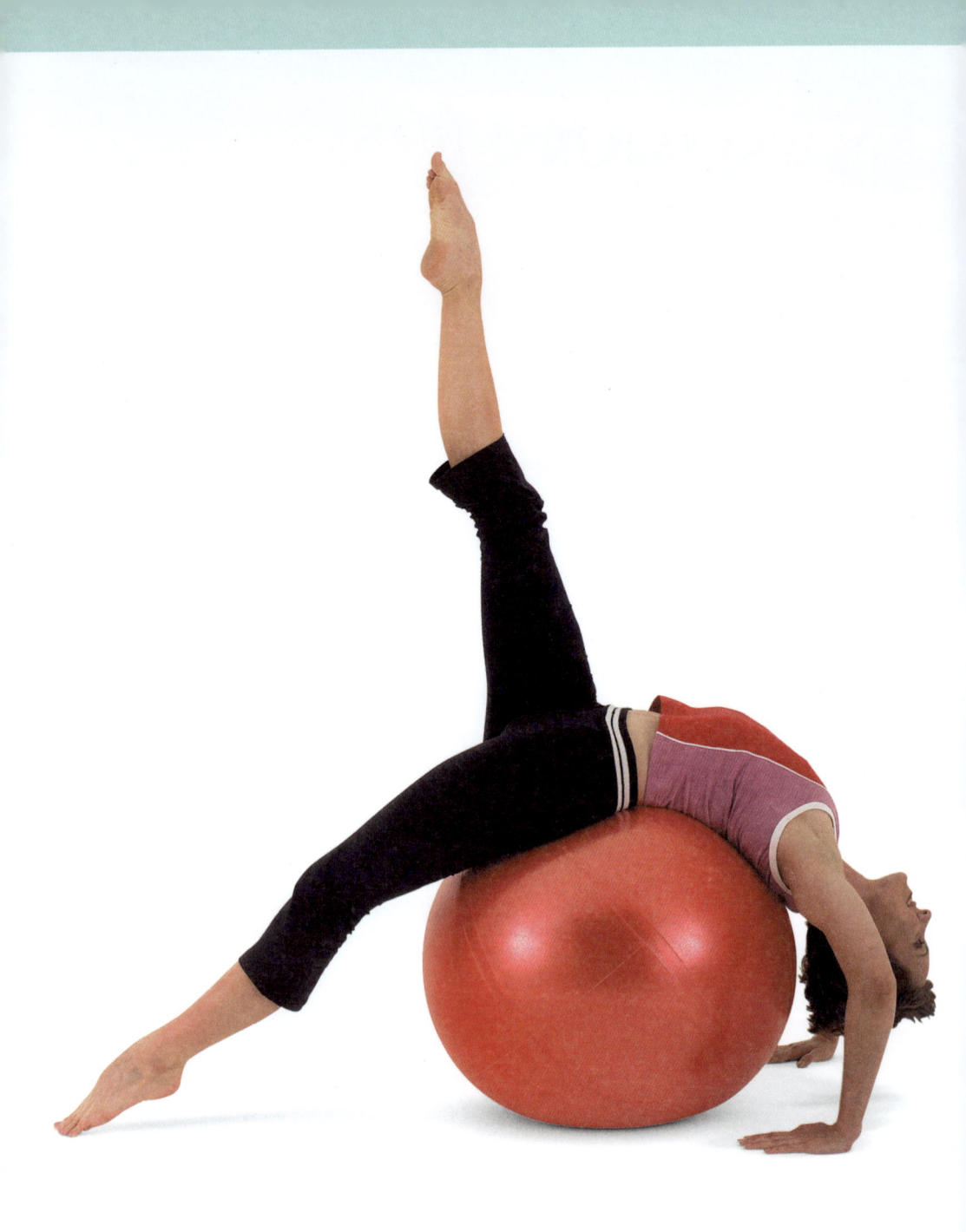

Introduction

The exercise ball, also known as the Swiss, therapy, physio, fitness, balance, gymnastic or stability ball, was originally used in Europe during the 1960s for the management of orthopedic and neurological problems. Physical therapists found that the ball's constant movement encouraged the individual to improve body and movement awareness, as well as call upon deeper layers of muscles necessary for overall joint stability, better posture and muscle balance. Use of the ball has extended from therapeutic applications to the sports medicine field and most recently to the general public in gyms and body-conditioning studios. The ball has become a versatile piece of exercise equipment. It can act as an aid to support the body weight and facilitate stretching, decrease stability at various angles to promote optimal strengthening of the whole body, or simply add new dimension and dynamics to any exercise regime. Strengthening the body in this way has been found to benefit the individual so that everyday activities or sporting endeavours are enhanced by improved movement mechanics, balanced strength of both sides of the body and faster reflex.

Exercising with the ball shares similarities with the principles behind the Pilates Method, which is a movement system that focuses on body alignment, balanced strength and movement control. The Method was developed by German-born Joseph Pilates in the early 1900s and he used his knowledge of the body to rehabilitate injured soldiers during World War I. He later opened an exercise studio in New York where he worked one-to-one with his clients, addressing their particular postural and structural needs. Pilates exercise sequences have endless scope for movement possibilities, ranging from a basic rehabilitative level to more advanced manoeuvres requiring greater athleticism and coordination. Many people worldwide enjoy the multi-dimensional qualities of the Pilates approach to exercise. The dynamics of the Method vary between studios and instructors, though the principles remain the same. It is a proven technique of developing and maintaining physical strength and mobility. It has a solid record of success with people of all ages and fitness levels and is adaptable to ever-evolving refinements in physical conditioning techniques.

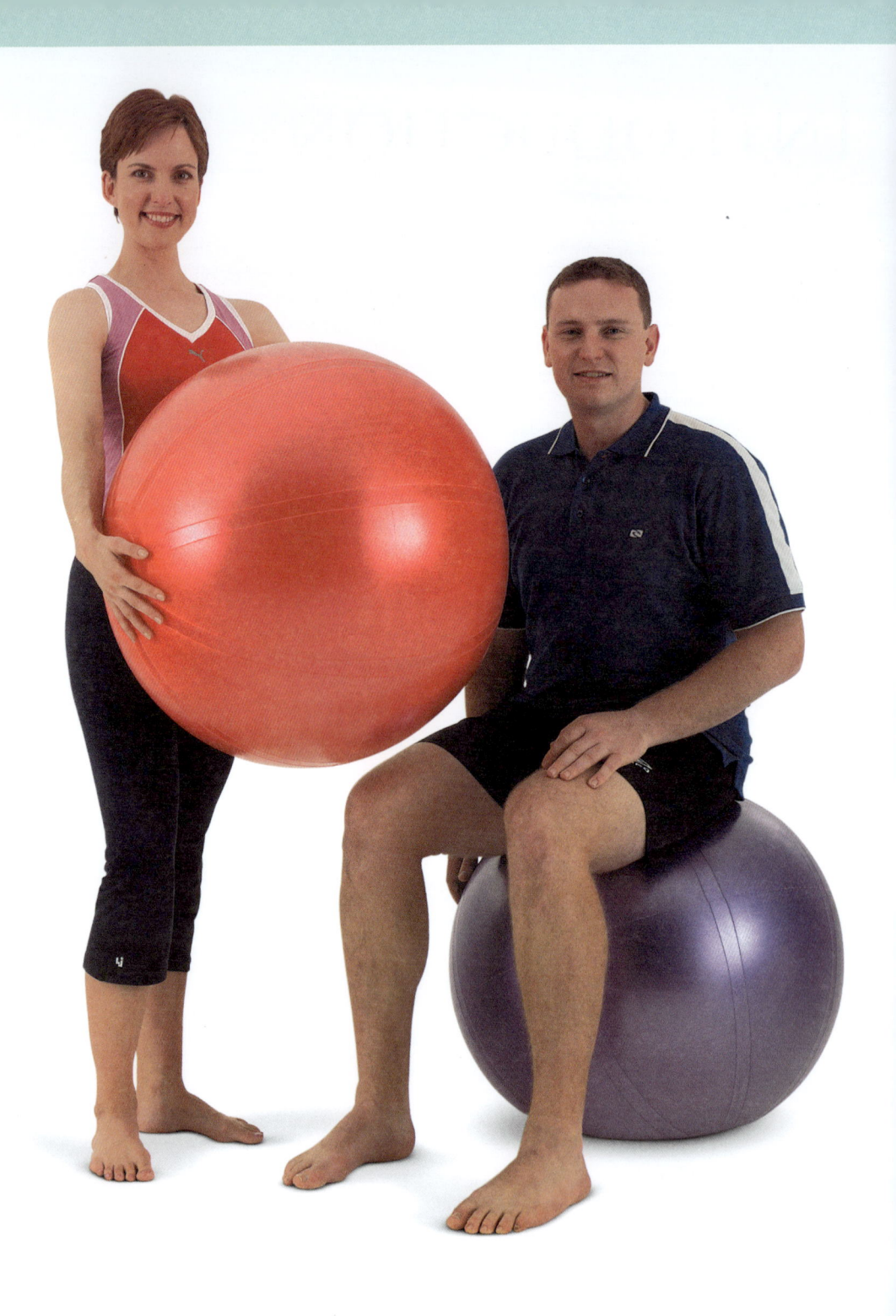

INTRODUCTION

The powerful fundamental principles of Pilates need to be understood and applied in order to achieve the most from practising this technique.

CONCENTRATION
Visualisation and mental focus are essential to gain muscle control.

CONTROL
Quality movement is most beneficial and less harmful to joints and muscles.

CENTRING
The abdomen, lower back, hips and buttocks, or the 'powerhouse', is the primary focus of strength, stability and 'core' control.

FLUIDITY
Graceful, flowing motion is required, with no static, jerky or rushed movements.

PRECISION
Purposeful movement with good body alignment develops better muscle patterns for everyday activities.

BREATHING
Applying a breathing pattern assists movement rhythm and control, as well as energising the whole system.

Blending the ball into a series of Pilates floor movements is a simple progression because the principles remain the same. The concept of torso stability and coordinating breath and abdominal control also apply when using the ball. As an unstable base, the ball can help the individual gain greater awareness of where they are in space, assist them in concentrating on the exact purpose of the exercise and especially focusing on a strong 'core'. Merely sitting on the ball has benefits for muscles otherwise unused, as well as promoting circulation with the constant adjustment of position needed to maintain an ideal posture. Balancing on the ball also encourages the muscles to release tension so that they can gain strength in a more effortless manner. The ball lends itself well to exercises that provide gentle stretching and movement of the spine in particular and Joseph Pilates used to declare that an individual is as young as his spine is flexible!

ESSENTIAL BALL • 8

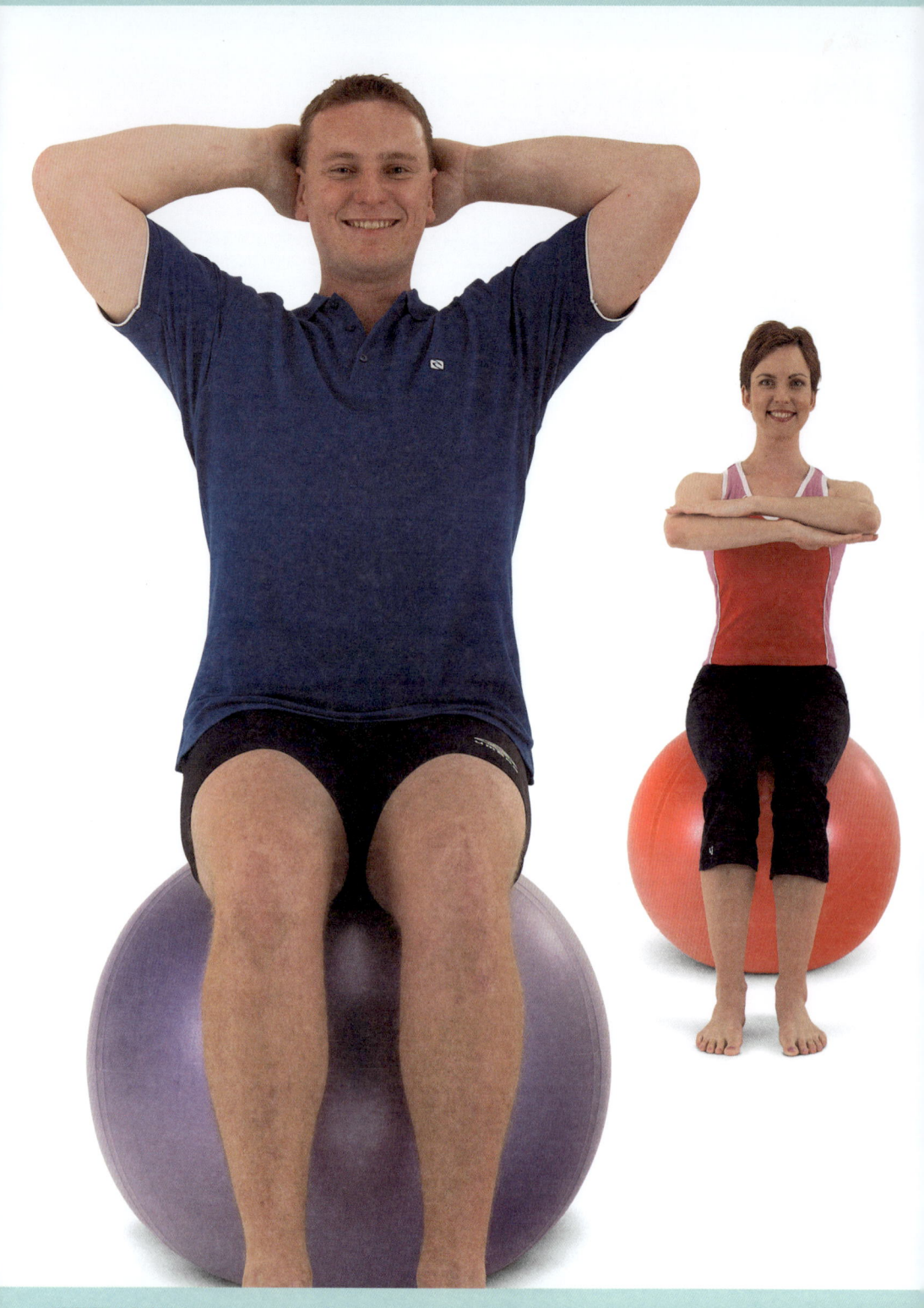

The Benefits

Now that many of us are finally steering away from the 'no pain, no gain' mentality of getting fit, patient measures can be taken to practise a more holistic way of developing control over movement, posture, physical vitality and, of course, the way we look. Incorporating the Pilates principles in your ball workout will enable you to develop overall body strength and tone rather than isolating larger muscle groups that are possibly already strong. We move about every day using our whole body and we should exercise with that in mind. Balancing on the unstable ball reinforces the focus of using the deep abdominal, back and pelvic muscles as the primary base of support for the torso. The 'centre', 'core' or 'powerhouse' will be strengthened and become more reliable for pelvic and spinal support during general daily activities. Having this area stronger and more stable will also enable you to have greater control over your limb movements. As the workout is mostly always moving—never static—further benefits include muscle endurance, greater coordination, poise and gracefulness.

Time spent exercising effectively is a wise investment in your physical future. Your exercise regime should provide you with functional results as well as being enjoyable and a 'break away' from your daily grind.

Exercising with the ball is one way to eradicate boredom, monotony or frenzy that many people associate with a workout. In order to exercise effectively for your health and perhaps reignite your enthusiasm for your efforts, you need to think of what you wish to achieve. Then, when you have an intention, you will exercise with purpose and over time you will accomplish positive results. Even if you already have an established fitness routine, it's possible to become stale which will result in loss of focus and concentration. Joseph Pilates believed that mindful intention behind a movement was the key to developing muscle control, correcting postural imbalances and restoring energy levels. The aim is intelligent exercise.

Anyone can grab an exercise ball and execute ten or more stomach 'crunches'. What makes this workout different is the inclusion of Pilates fundamentals. The technique is so precise and focused that correct execution becomes a physical discipline much like dance or martial arts. This physical training is unique with its emphasis on lengthening muscles while strengthening them, stabilising the lumbar spine and pelvis while movement of the limbs and upper torso is fluid, and controlled breathing which provides a rhythm and facilitates deep abdominal connection.

Practical Matters

Every person has different needs when exercising and you should aim for the ideal posture and muscular balance for your own physique. Primarily, always ensure that you keep your deep abdominal muscles lifted and drawn in towards your lower back. Never grip your muscles. Think of them like sponges that you gently squeeze, press, stretch or lengthen. How you perform each movement is the essence of what Pilates body conditioning is—understand the aim of the exercise, focus on the part of you that is stable and the part that is moving smoothly. Work your body from the core out, instead of relying on the superficial muscle layers. Remember that there is no real benefit in dozens of thoughtless repetitions in a vain attempt to achieve a beautiful body. 'Less is more', with a maximum of 6–10 repetitions being sufficient for each exercise. Be consistent with a slower pace with greater attention to accuracy and control. Practising your ball workout three to four times a week is good, depending upon your other activities, though certainly try to spend time daily on a few of the initial exercises that will reinforce the principles for you. This sensible approach to your body-conditioning regime is like 'building blocks'—you will gradually add dimension to your exercises, layer upon layer, developing your ability to perform movements with ease and grace.

If you have an injury—past or present—or if you are pregnant or post-surgery, it is strongly recommended that you consult your doctor or physical therapist before embarking on any exercise program. Remember that some of the following exercises may be unsuitable for your body and you may have to modify them, or avoid them.

Requirements

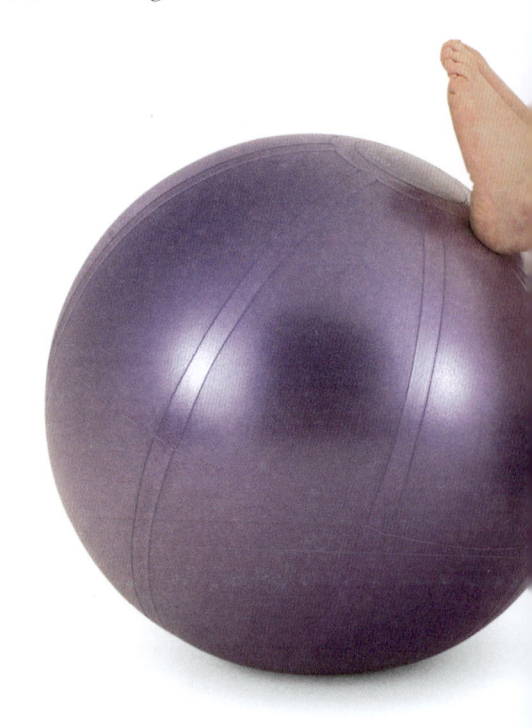

Quality exercise balls are available through various distributors, in particular medical supply and sporting good outlets. Ideally choose one regarded as 'burst-resistant' for greater safety, durability and shape integrity over time. They are generally available in a variety of sizes and colours. The appropriate size for you is one that allows your hip joints to be angled slightly higher than your knees when you are seated on the ball. A ball too small will disturb your neutral spinal and pelvic alignment and one too large will become too difficult to control during your workout. Balls are inflatable with various pumps. The first time you inflate your ball don't fill it completely and let it settle for some hours before increasing the firmness. A softer ball will give you more support and stability; if inflated too hard it may be uncomfortable and too difficult for you to balance on.

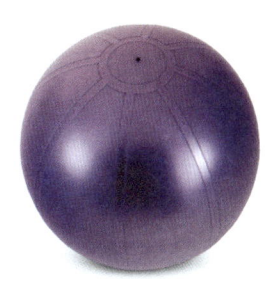

Wear clothing that is comfortable and won't restrict your movement. Exercise on a mat for some spinal support and when you are lying on the ball ensure that it doesn't slip on the floor surface.

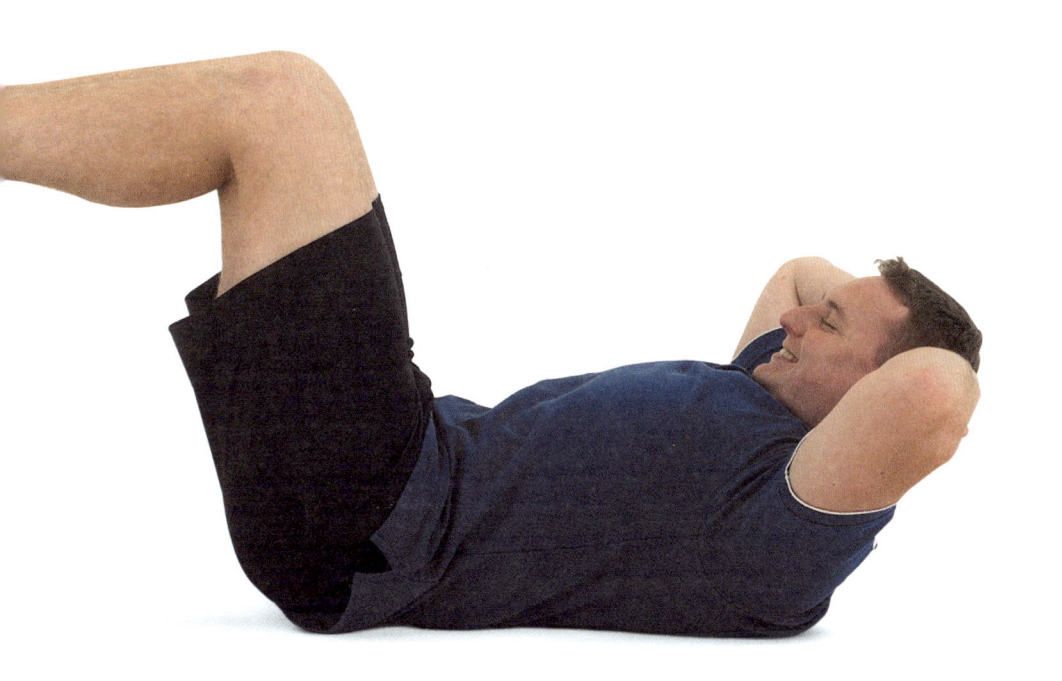

Centring & Breathing

The following three concepts should become a central focus for you throughout your ball workout. They are the foundation of the Pilates principles and will aid you in correct and intended execution of each exercise.

Neutral Pelvis Position

The pelvis is a base of support for the spine and when it moves there are direct repercussions for the spinal curves. When the pelvis tilts forward or backward the position of the lower back, in particular, changes. Ongoing clinical research into the prevention and management of back pain demonstrates that maintaining the natural curvature of the spine is necessary while developing strength and endurance of the deep abdominal and paraspinal muscles associated with achieving 'core stability'. While practising Pilates and ball exercises a 'neutral pelvis' position is the ideal basis for correct spinal alignment. This position is easy to find when lying on your back if you relax your hip and back muscles so that no tilt of the pelvis occurs. Your two hip bones (iliac crests) and your pubic bone all form a parallel level with the floor. Think of the back of your pelvis as an anchor point while on the floor, so that you develop a feeling of stability through your centre. When sitting, standing or lying on your back, side or front, you should be able to develop the same corset-type stability with this alignment intact. When sitting, be right on top of your sitting bones to help you find your Neutral Pelvis position—you'd feel these if you were to sit on a hard surface, as they are the lowest boney protrusions of the pelvis.

Correct Abdominals

The Pilates approach to abdominal strengthening was originally aimed at achieving greater support for the back and pelvis. Joseph Pilates' technique of maintaining a stable pelvis and lumbar spine while flattening the abdomen firmly during leg and upper torso movement corresponds with current methods of 'core stabilisation'. The action of the abdominals during this process must entail a broadening and flattening sensation of the lower abdominal region while also lifting or drawing up the muscles of the pelvic floor, which support the bladder. Typical expressions of such instructions during a Pilates workout include 'scooping', 'hollowing', 'navel to spine', 'draw in and up' or 'zipping', among others. The idea is being able to visualise internally how your lower abdominals are acting in order to help stabilise your pelvis and reinforce your spine. It is appropriate for everyone to focus on strengthening the deeper muscles of the abdomen so that other muscles—in particular, hip and lower back muscles—don't become dominant and overtight.

Breath Control

How you breathe while executing the exercises will determine how well you develop muscle control and stamina. The

Pilates technique of breathing requires you to breathe laterally, which means expanding the side and back of the lower ribcage while taking in air. This will enable you to still focus on the abdominal muscles drawing inward and upward toward your spine. Purposeful breathing throughout exercising will also create an even working pace and assist you in maintaining full control of each movement. You should not over-emphasise deep breathing, but simply be aware of this breathing technique while you learn to coordinate accurate movements with correct abdominal patterning. Breathing should be calming and assist you in releasing tension from the muscles you don't need to use while you focus on improving your posture and general wellbeing.

Preparatory Note

Embody these three basic postural essentials and gradually learn to coordinate movement while managing these subtle changes. Start to become aware of the alignment of your body as a whole structure—your Neutral Pelvis position, the natural curves of your spine, your hip, knee and ankle joints in line, your shoulder blades gently held back and flat against your ribs, your chin gently lowered and the back of your neck lengthened upward. This will help you understand the intentions behind the Pilates principles and the Simply Ball Workout. More importantly, these ideas should provide you with a basis for restoring posture and balance to your everyday life.

Breathing Exercise

Purpose To establish the three basic postural concepts while lying on the floor, or seated on the ball. Create an awareness of where your pelvis and spine are positioned in a neutral alignment and learn how to coordinate a lateral breathing technique with a strong sense of your deep abdominal muscles supporting your back. Begin every exercise with this same preparation and incorporate these principles throughout your ball workout. This practice will soon become second nature as you focus all your movements around a strong and stable centre.

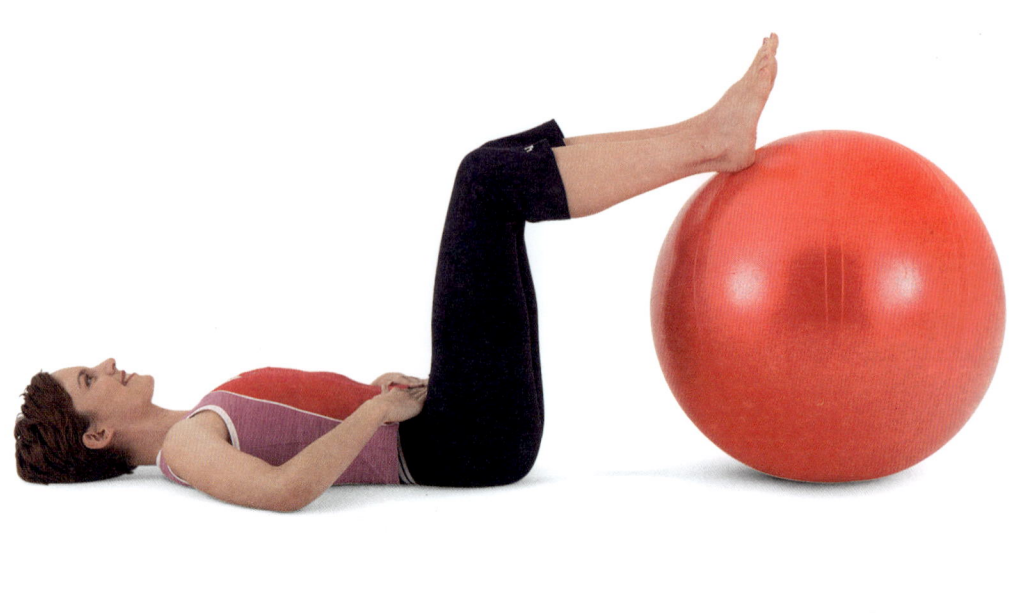

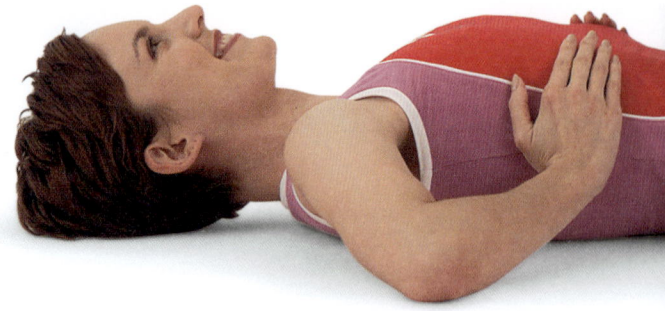

1. Lie on your back with your heels on the ball, knees and ankles slightly apart. Position your knees vertically above your hips and place your hands on your lower abdomen.

2. Establish a calm breathing pace, just as you would normally breathe, while maintaining an awareness of your Neutral Pelvis position and relaxed neck and shoulders. Breathe in, count four. Breathe out, count four. Repeat for a moment.

3. Now, continue the lateral breathing pattern and begin scooping your lower abdominals deep toward a central spot in your mid-lower back. You may place your hands on your ribs to be more aware of the sideways breathing action. Maintain the lift of your pelvic floor each inhale and re-emphasise the navel-to-spine action with each exhale.

4. Then practise this posture and lateral breathing pattern while seated on the ball. Make sure you are sitting on your 'sitting bones' rather than being too far back on the ball and allowing the backs of your thighs to bear your body weight.

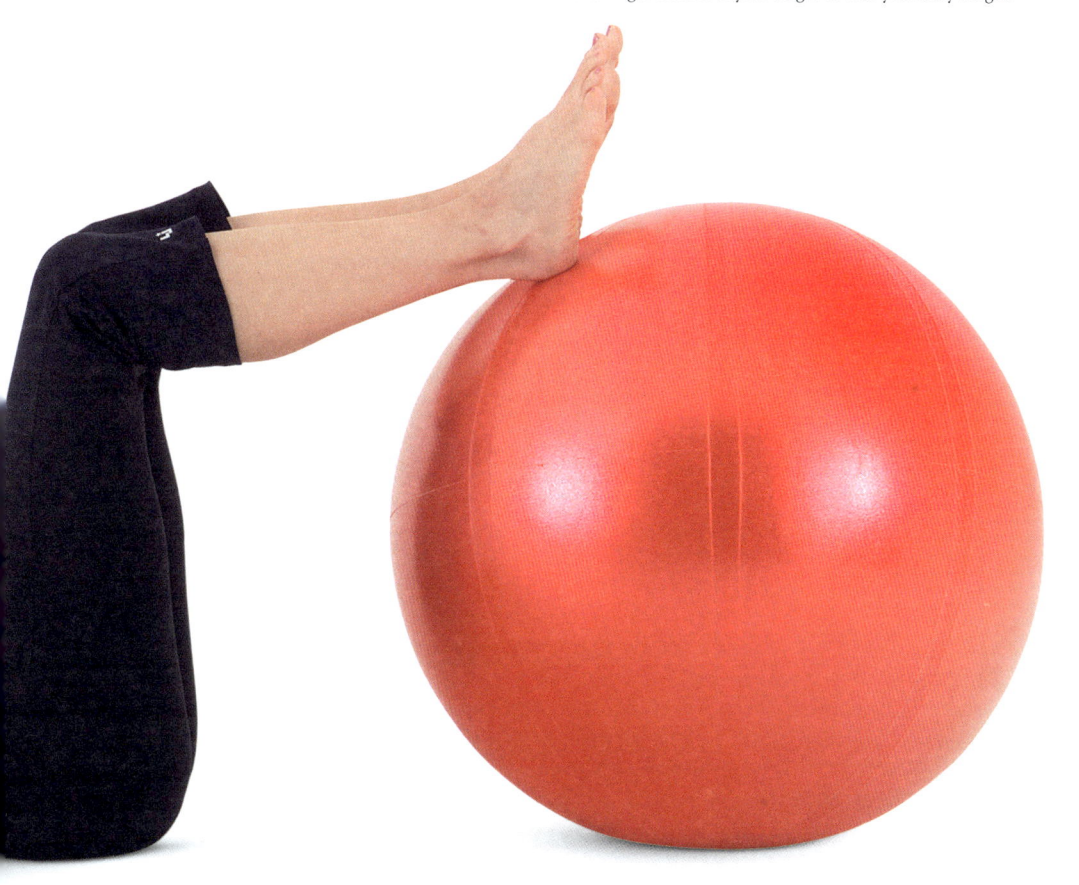

Posture Awareness & Abdominal Preparation

Purpose To establish a neutral alignment of the pelvis and spine while seated on the ball and learn balance and efficient posture control so the body's musculature does not overwork. Also, incorporating small movements of the lower and upper torso for abdominal warm-up.

Seated Balance

1. Sit on the ball as though you are seated in a straight-backed chair, with your feet no more than hip-width apart. Maintain a Neutral Pelvis position, draw your navel toward the spine and lengthen your waist. Feel as though you're weightless and buoyant, so you don't slouch into the ball. Try to limit the use of your feet and legs to stabilise your body.

2. Lift one thigh as you inhale and lower it as you exhale. Concentrate on the stability of your opposite hip and waist. Alternate legs so you become accustomed to transferring your weight while thinking of your centre. Remember not to lose your 'straight-backed chair' posture.

3. Repeat 10 times, alternating legs. Place your hands behind your head for further challenge.

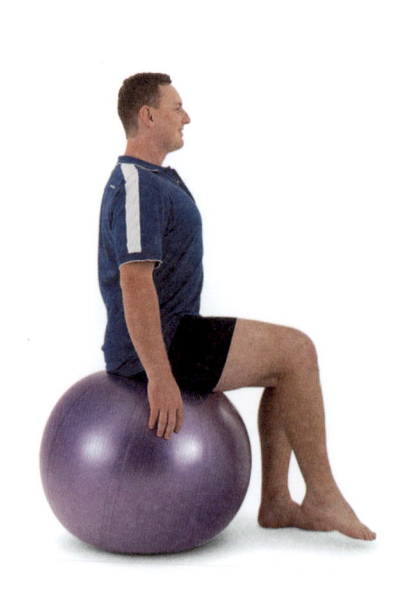

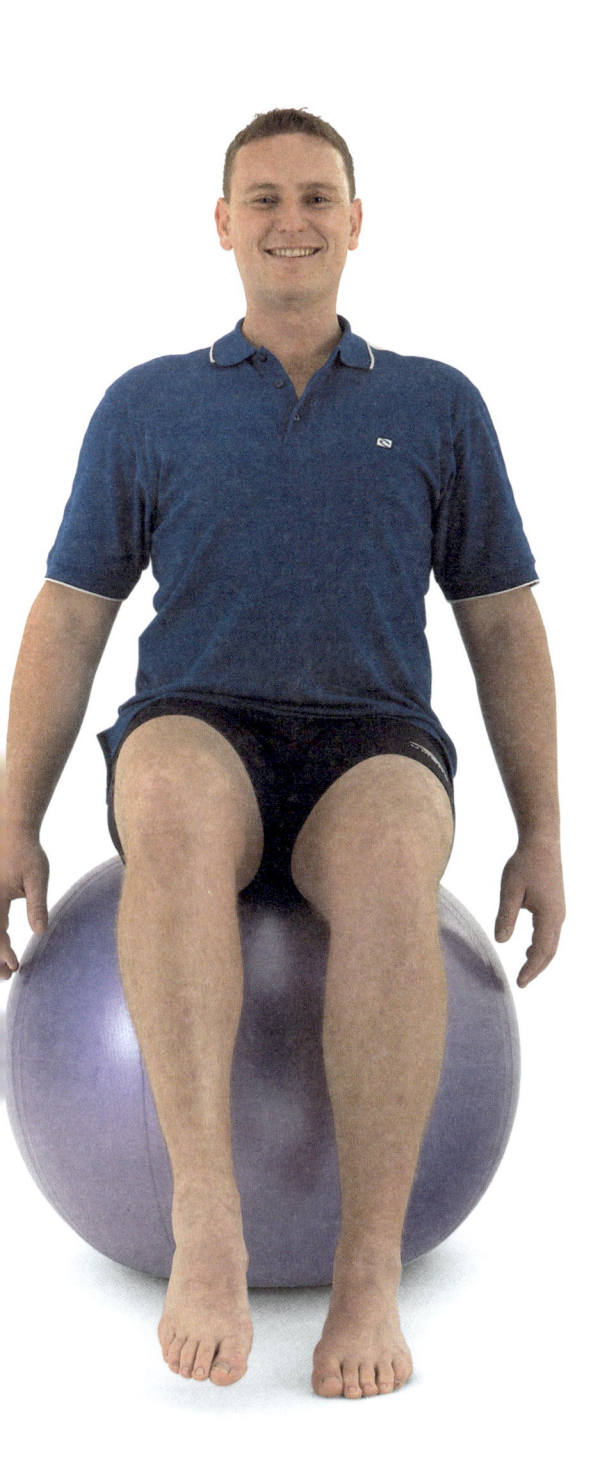

Note

Try to find your sitting bones—the hard 'bottom bones' you would be aware of if you were to sit on a hard surface. Think of these as your 'feet', when you're not standing on your feet. So, make sure that you distribute your body weight down through your sitting bones, rather than through the back of your thighs.

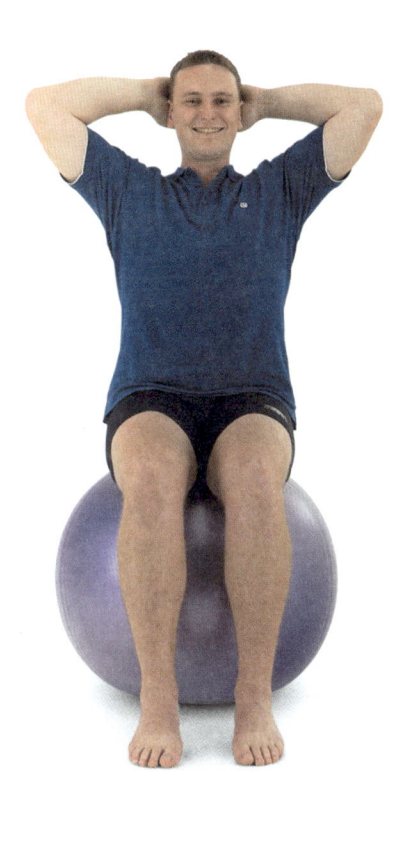

Posture Awareness & Abdominal Preparation

(continued)

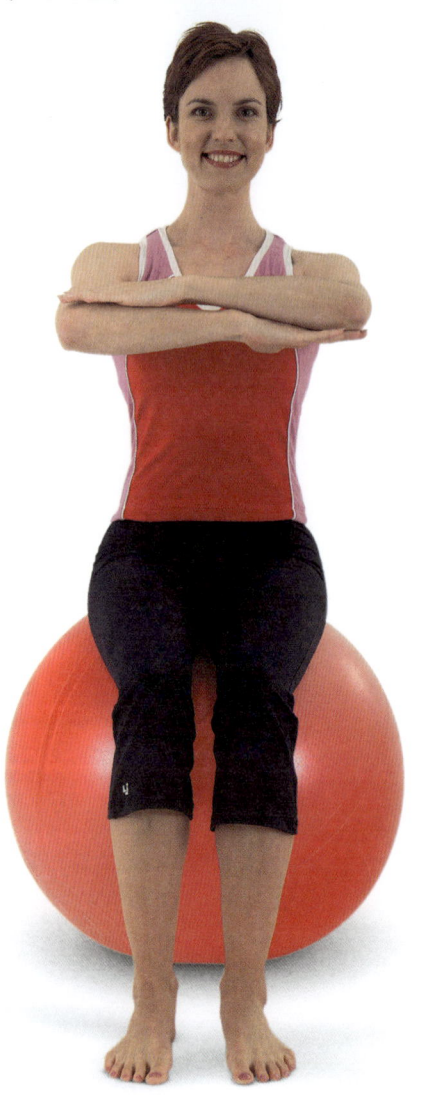

Pelvic Tilt

1 Inhale, lengthen your lower ribs up away from your hips and scoop your abdominals firmly toward your spine. Maintain your natural spinal curvature.

2 As you exhale, further scoop your abdominals and roll your pelvis back into the ball. Keep your ribcage fairly still in space as you roll your tail under, rounding your lower back.

3 Hold still as you inhale—remember your lateral breathing pattern—and reverse the roll as you exhale so as to resume an erect posture. Lengthen the front and back of your waist area equally so you don't end up over-extending your spine.

4 Repeat 4–6 times.

5 Following your last repetition, roll your pelvis under and walk your feet forward so you can lie back on the ball to prepare for Chest Lift on the Ball.

ESSENTIAL BALL • 19

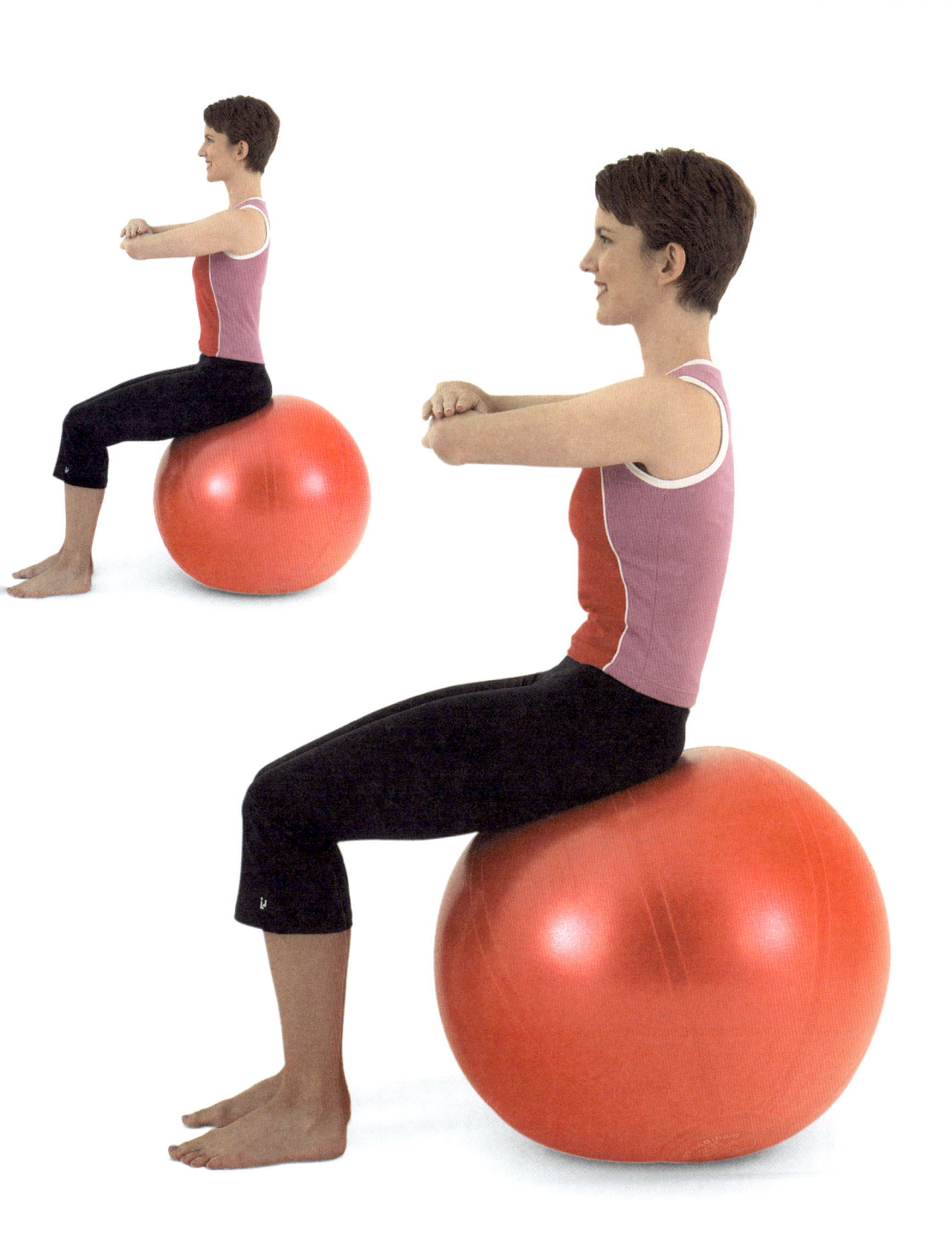

Posture Awareness & Abdominal Preparation

(continued)

Chest Lift on the Ball

1 Make sure that your back, from the tips of your shoulder blades to the back of your pelvis is in contact with the ball. Place your hands behind your head and have your feet no more than hip-width apart to promote good knee alignment.

2 With your hands supporting the head and neck lean back partially, scoop your abdominals and inhale to prepare. Imagine aiming your lower abdominals towards the back of your pelvis—a couple of inches below 'belt-line'.

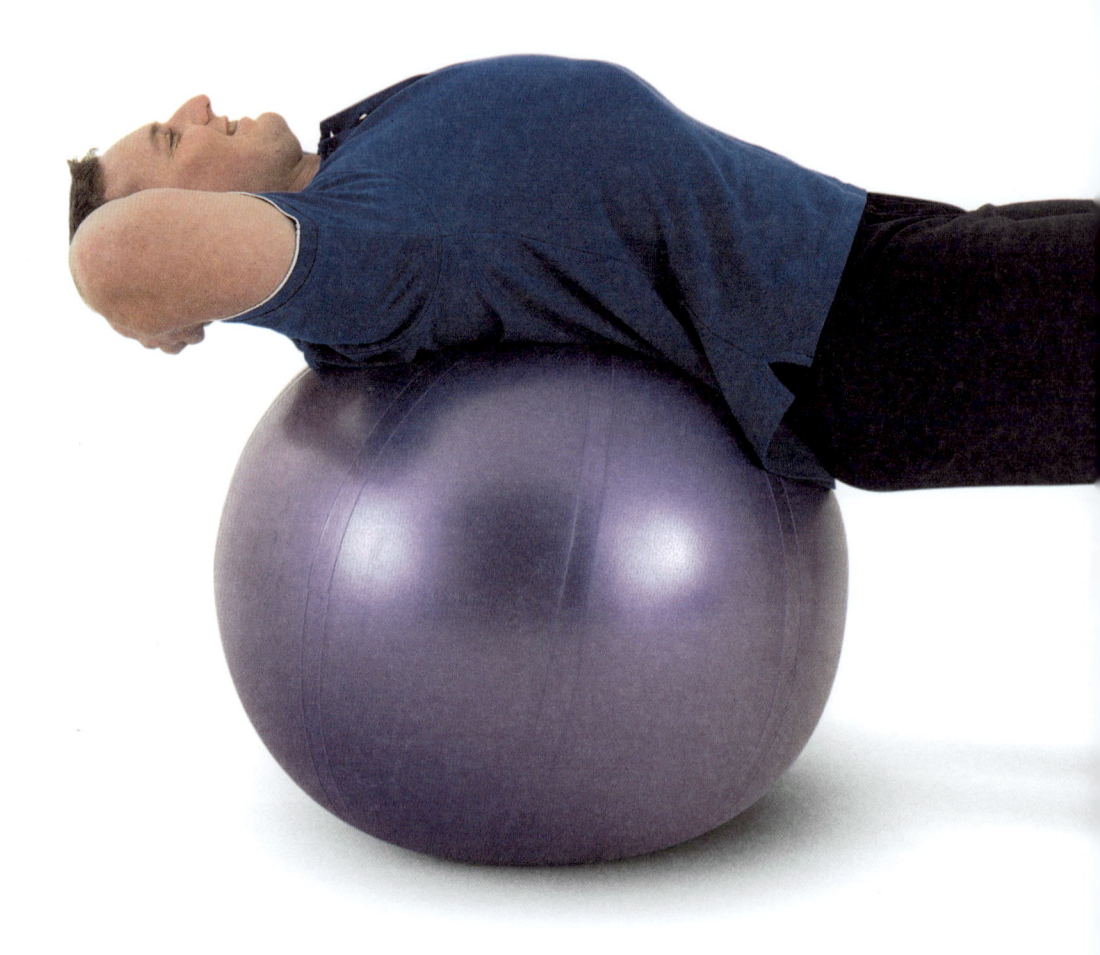

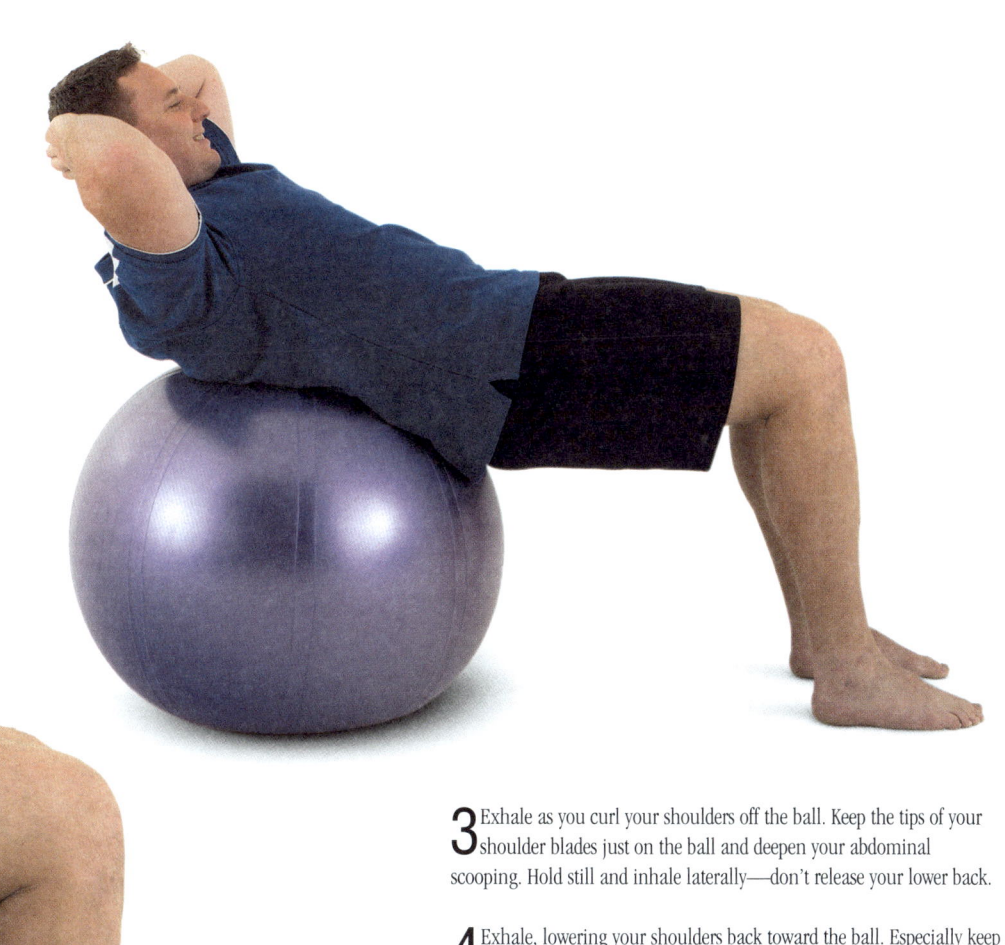

3 Exhale as you curl your shoulders off the ball. Keep the tips of your shoulder blades just on the ball and deepen your abdominal scooping. Hold still and inhale laterally—don't release your lower back.

4 Exhale, lowering your shoulders back toward the ball. Especially keep your back and abdominals strong here. Inhale, prepare again.

5 Repeat 4–6 times.

6 Change the breathing pattern. Exhale as you curl and inhale as you lower, so there is no stopping and coordination is challenged. Keep the lower half of your torso absolutely still and strong while the shoulder girdle is free to move. Remember breathing laterally will assist you in scooping ever-so-strong lower abdominals.

7 Repeat 4–6 times.

Abdominal Strengthening & Pelvic Stability

Purpose To develop a strong and stable mid-section. This is the essence of the Pilates method, executing various limb and upper torso movement to work the deep abdominal muscles and challenge the stability of the pelvis and lumbar spine.

Leg Pull

1. Lie on your back with your heels on the ball, slightly apart, and knees vertically aligned with your hips. Maintain a Neutral Pelvis position and place your hands on your hips. Breathe laterally and scoop your abdominals.

2. As you inhale allow the ball to roll away, not completely straightening the legs. Maintain your abdominal bracing and back stability.

3. Draw the ball back toward you as you exhale. Emphasise each drawing in action of the legs, ensuring your abdominals reinforce the spine in its neutral position.

4. Repeat 4–6 times.

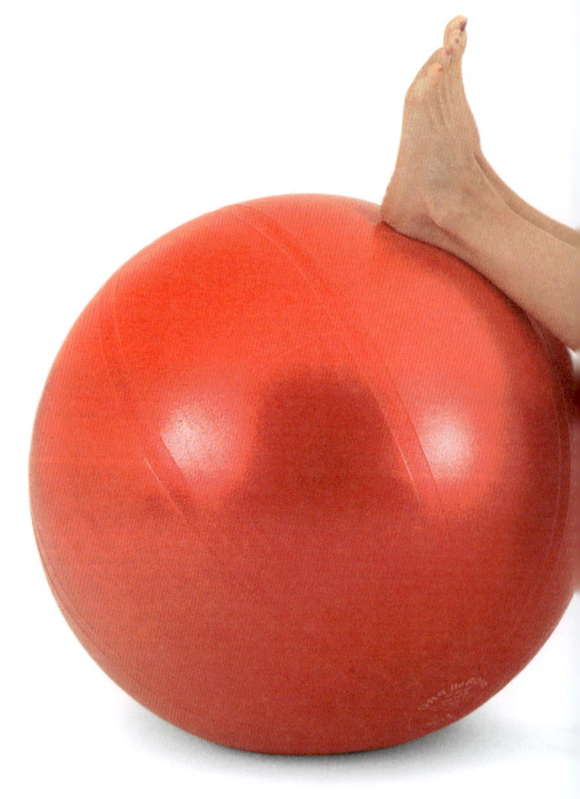

PROGRESSION

Keep a stable back as you now move double time—inhale for the 'in' and 'out' movement and exhale as you do the next 'in' and 'out'. So, the legs may move a little quicker, but your breathing stays calm and controlled—as do your abdominals, scooping straight to your spine. Try to have a mental picture of what body part is strong and still and what is free to move. This is a key fundamental in learning how to embody Pilates principles. Repeat 4–6 times

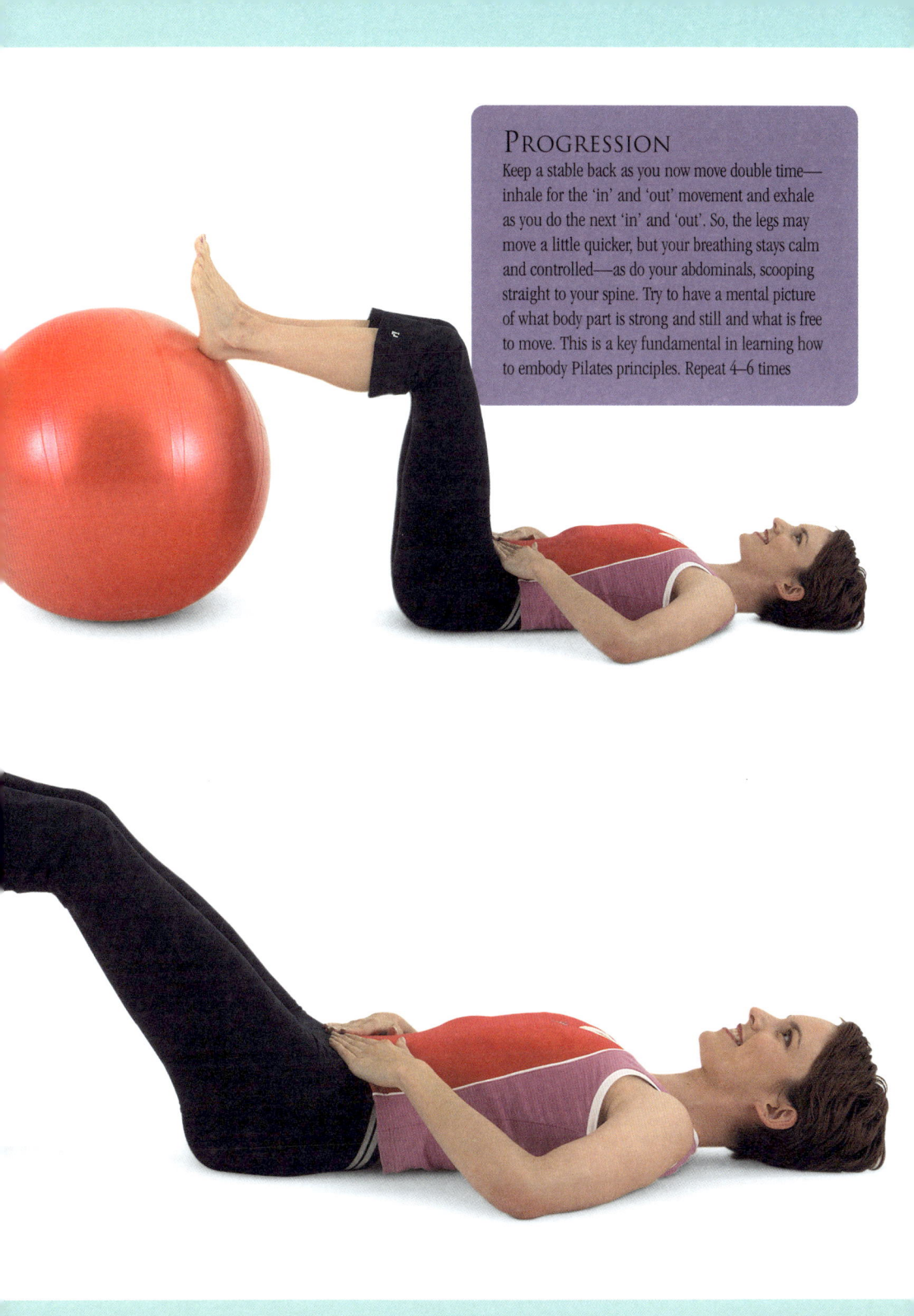

Abdominal Strengthening & Pelvic Stability

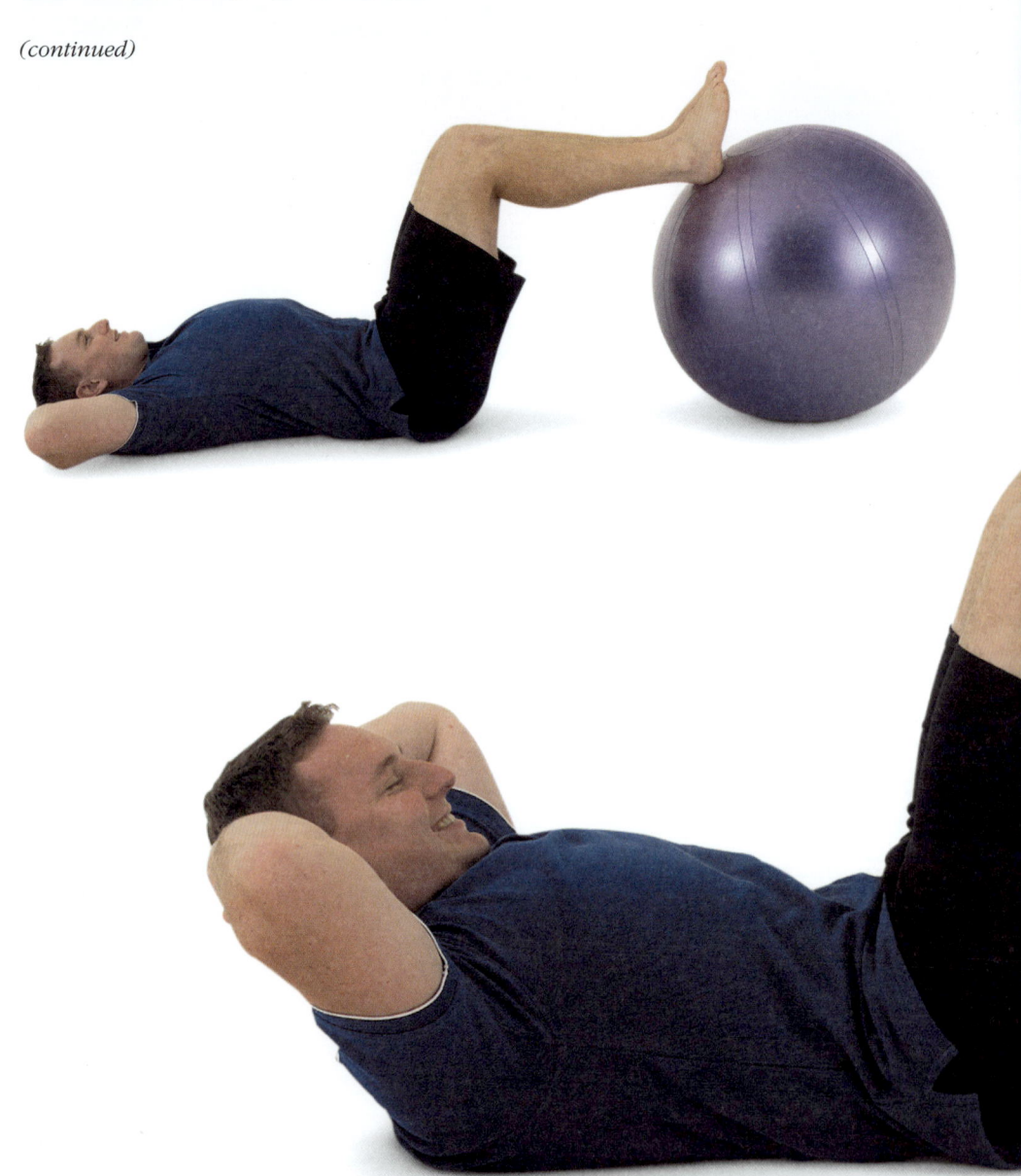

(continued)

Chest Lift

1 Begin as for Leg Pull and place your hands under your head and neck. Breathe in, focusing navel to spine. Use this preparation at the beginning of all your abdominal exercises.

2 Exhale as you curl your head, neck and shoulders just clear of the floor. Emphasise your scooping abdominals and stable back and pelvis.

3 Inhale laterally as you lower back to the floor with control. There should be absolutely no release of the lower back as you lie back to the floor. Remember that the role of your abdominals is to reinforce the front side of your spine.

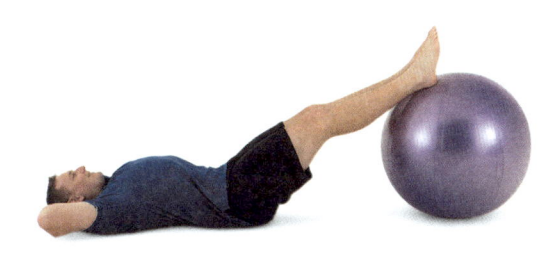

4 Repeat 4–6 times.

Progression

Begin with your legs extended away from you and as you curl your head and shoulders off the floor pull both legs toward you. Repeat 4–6 times.

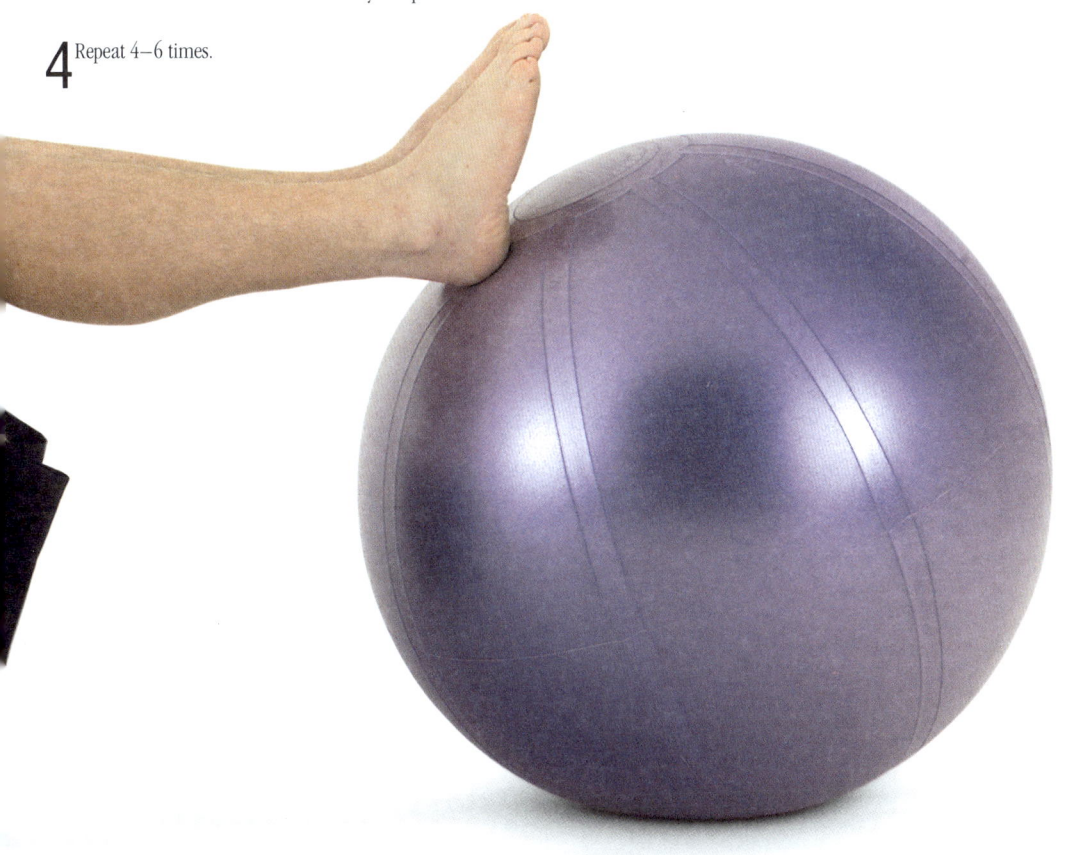

ESSENTIAL BALL • 25

Abdominal Strengthening & Pelvic Stability

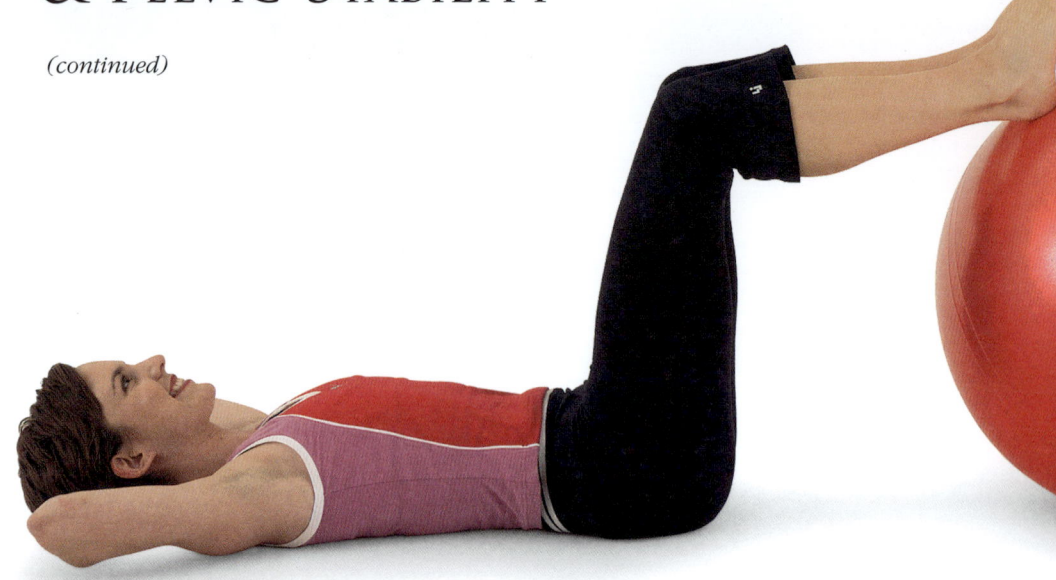

(continued)

Oblique Lifts

1. Begin as for Chest Lift. Inhale as you prepare your abdominals. Stabilise the pelvis and lower back.

2. As you exhale lift the head and shoulders, rotating your upper torso so that you aim one shoulder to the opposite hip. Maintain a stable Neutral Pelvis and focus on the side of the waist that you twist towards. Imagine 'pinning' your waist to the floor.

3. Inhale as you lower—keep your abdominals scooping all the while as this is essentially a preparation for your next repetition.

4. Alternate sides, 4–6 times.

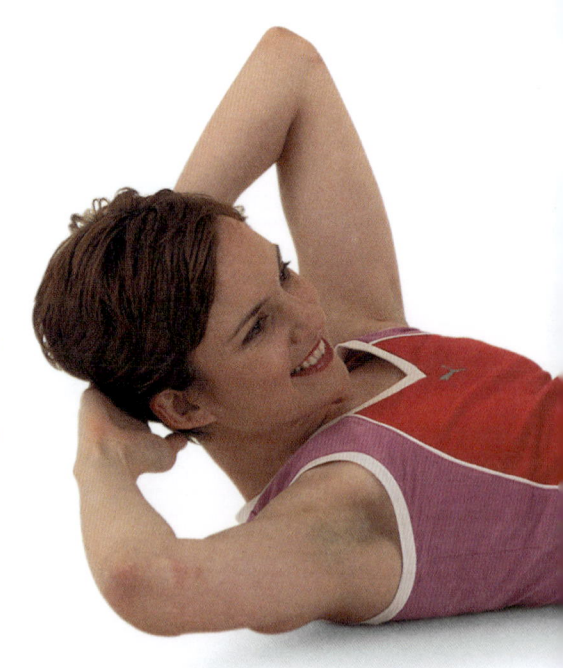

PROGRESSION
Begin with your legs extended and add the Leg Pull as you did with Chest Lift. Ensure that your legs don't come closer to you than a 90-degree angle with your hips. Alternate sides for 4 repetitions.

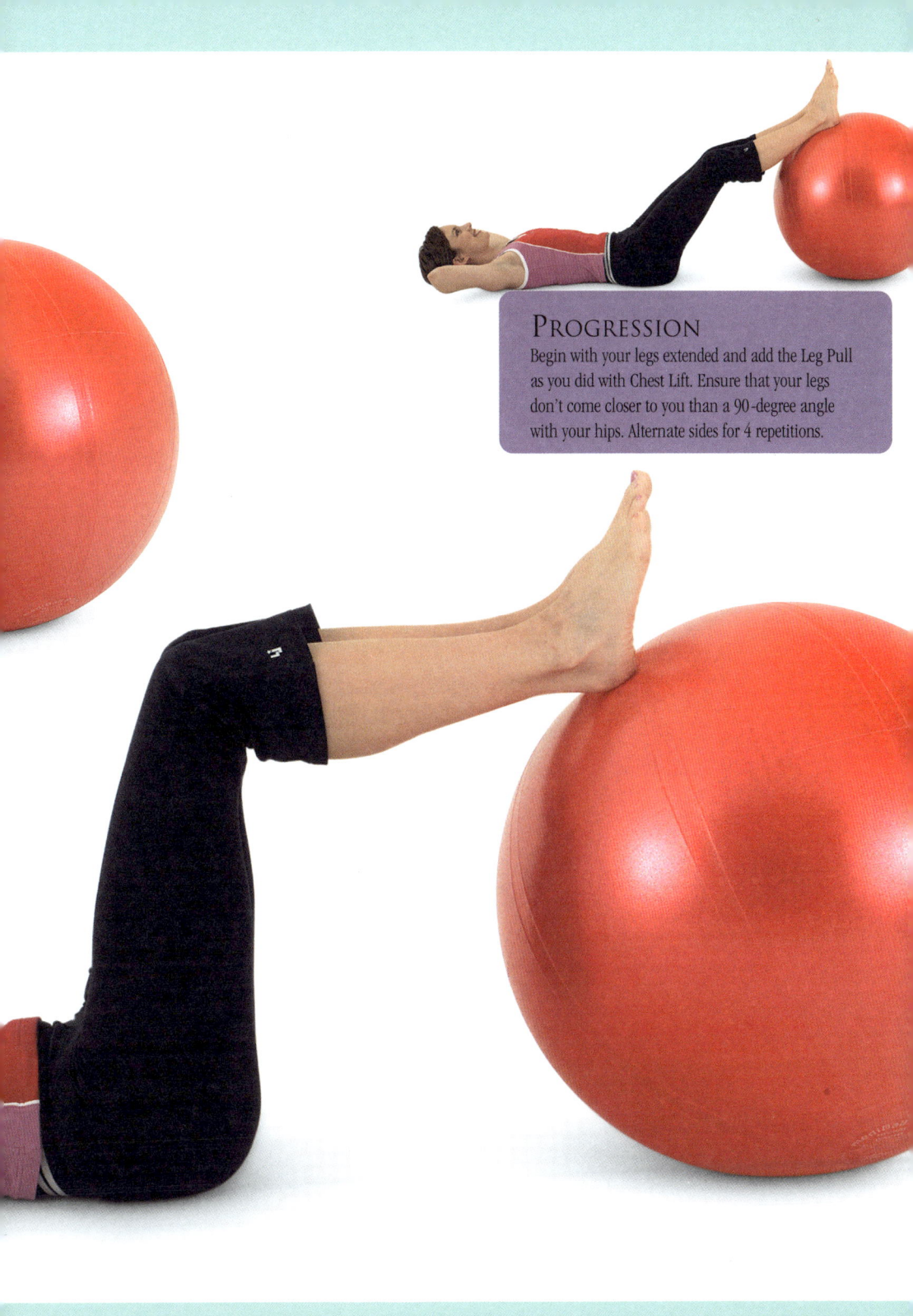

ESSENTIAL BALL • 27

Abdominal Strengthening & Pelvic Stability

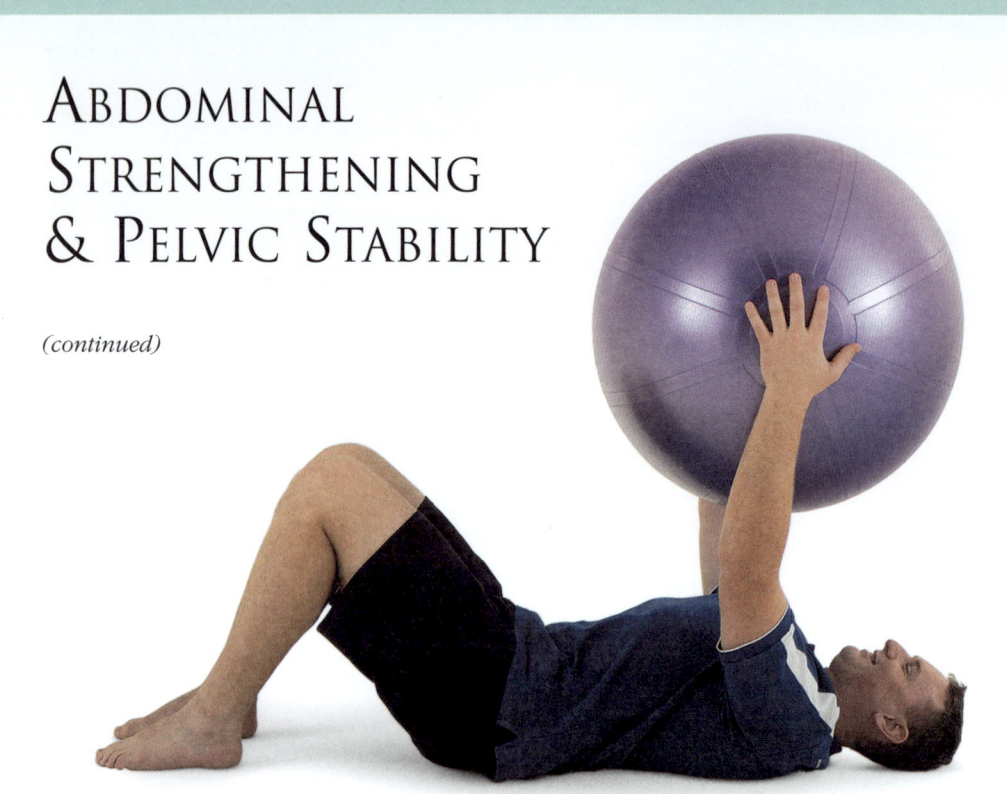

(continued)

Roll Up Prep

1 Begin lying on your back with your legs bent, knees and feet slightly apart. Reach your arms to the ceiling and lightly squeeze the ball between your hands. Draw your shoulders down and secure the back and pelvis by scooping your abdominals. Breathe in.

2 Exhale, lifting your head, neck and shoulders and reaching the ball beyond your knees. Focus on your abdominals—imagine your navel-to-spine action scooping right up under your ribs. Inhale, hold strong and still.

3 Exhale as you roll back to the floor with control, pressing your abdominals inward and upward.
Finish with the ball reaching for the ceiling.

4 Repeat 5 times.

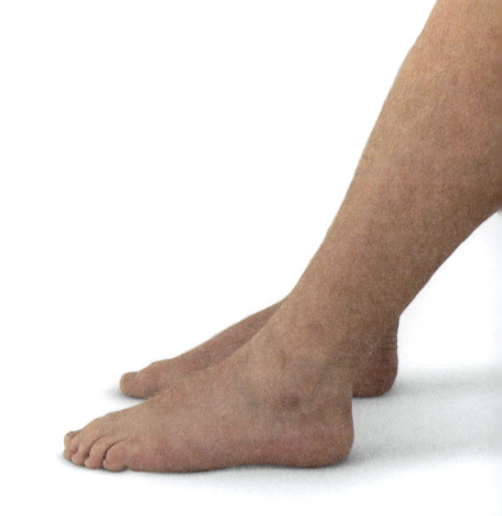

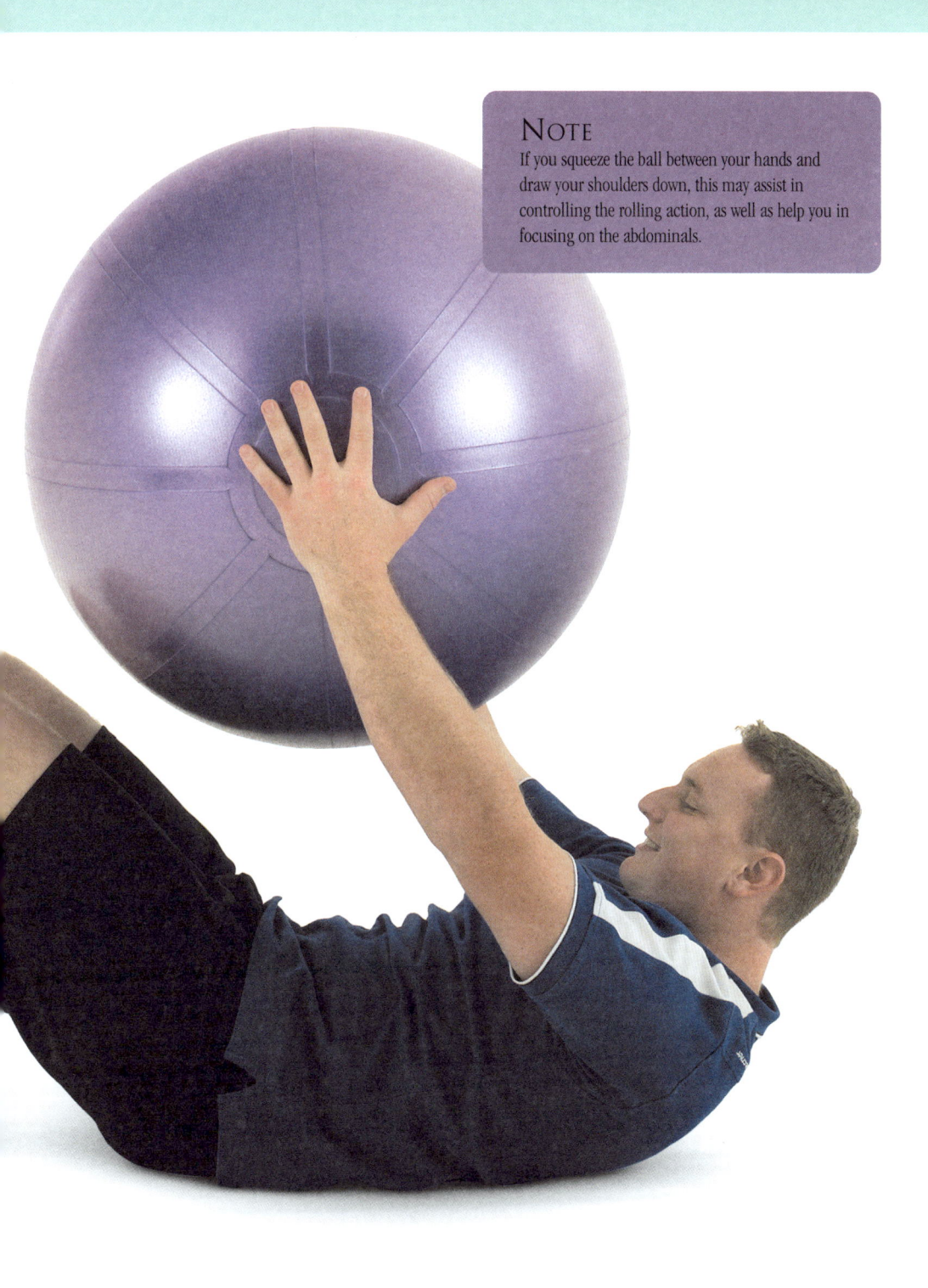

Note

If you squeeze the ball between your hands and draw your shoulders down, this may assist in controlling the rolling action, as well as help you in focusing on the abdominals.

ESSENTIAL BALL • 29

Abdominal Strengthening & Pelvic Stability

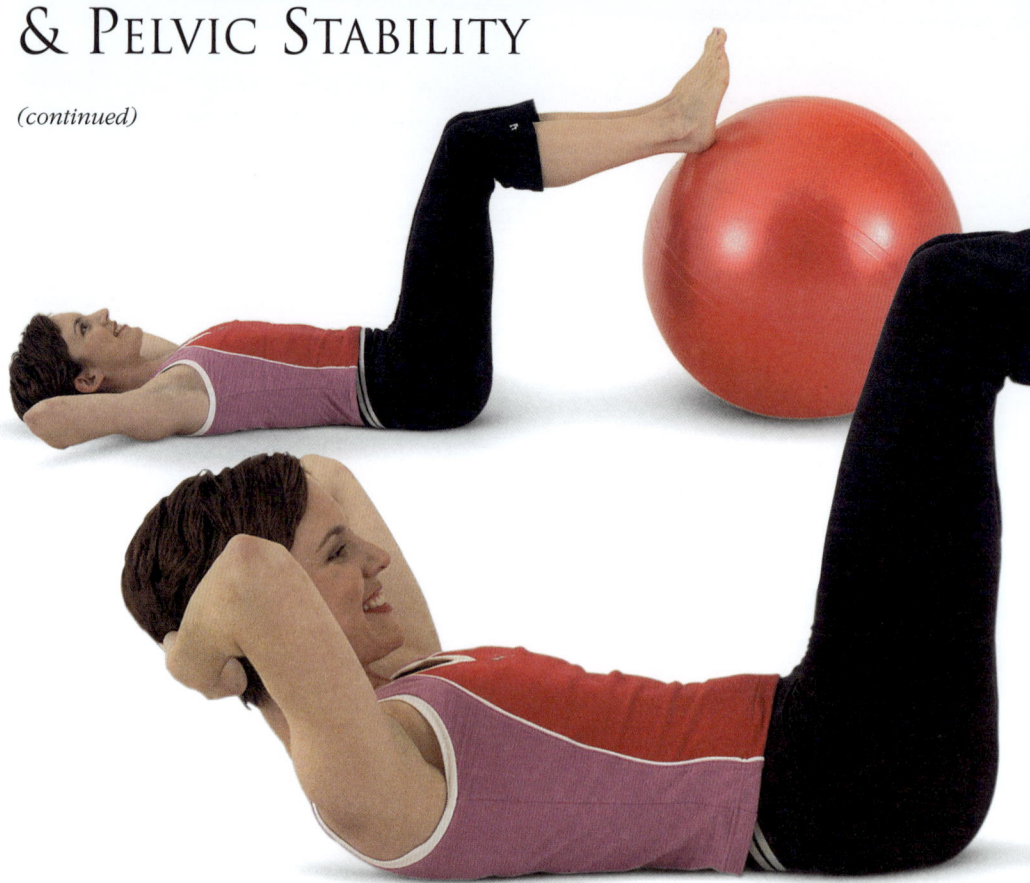

(continued)

Double Leg Stretch

1 Begin lying on your back with your feet on the ball, knees bent and aligned over your hips. Place your hands behind your head and neck. Start the exercise as though doing a Chest Lift. Inhale, prepare.

2 Curl your head, neck and shoulders off the floor as you exhale. Scoop your abdominals.

3 Inhale, push the ball away and exhale as you draw it back toward you. Repeat the leg pull 4 times in all, then inhale to hold still and strong.

4 Exhale as you lower your head and shoulders. Maintain constant control of your back, pelvis and abdominals—try not to focus primarily on the ball.

5 Repeat all for 2 sets.

Progression

Begin in the same position, though place your hands on your knees. Lift your head and shoulders on the exhale and when you inhale, push your legs out and extend your arms up by the sides of your head, so that toes and fingers reach in opposite directions. Take great care not to release your back and stomach. Emphasise the exhale, when you circle the arms and 'pull' your knees and hands back together. Try to imagine your abdominals do the 'pull'—your centre stays absolutely strong and the back of your pelvis remains anchored to the floor. Repeat all for 2 sets.

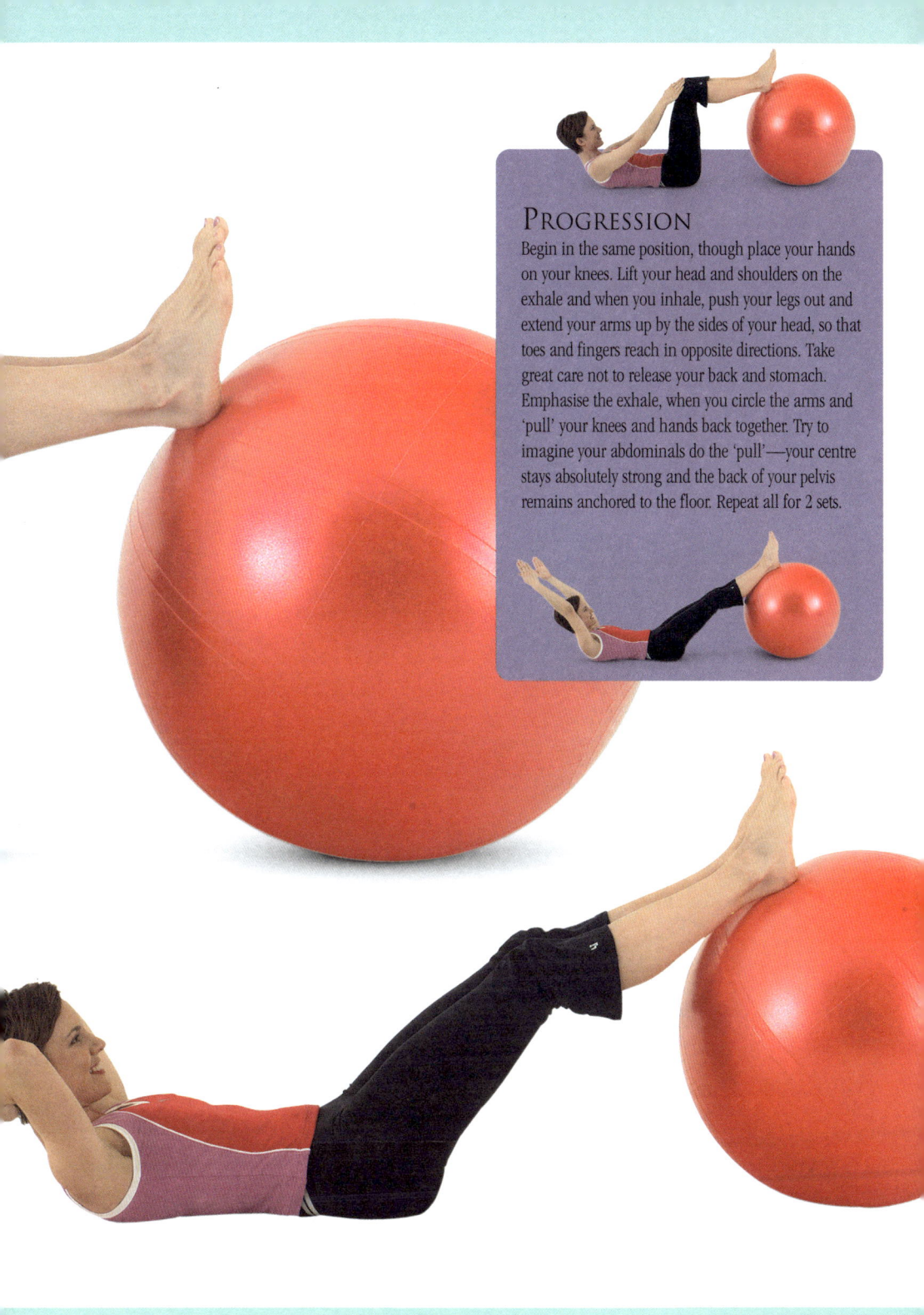

ESSENTIAL BALL • 31

Abdominal Strengthening & Pelvic Stability

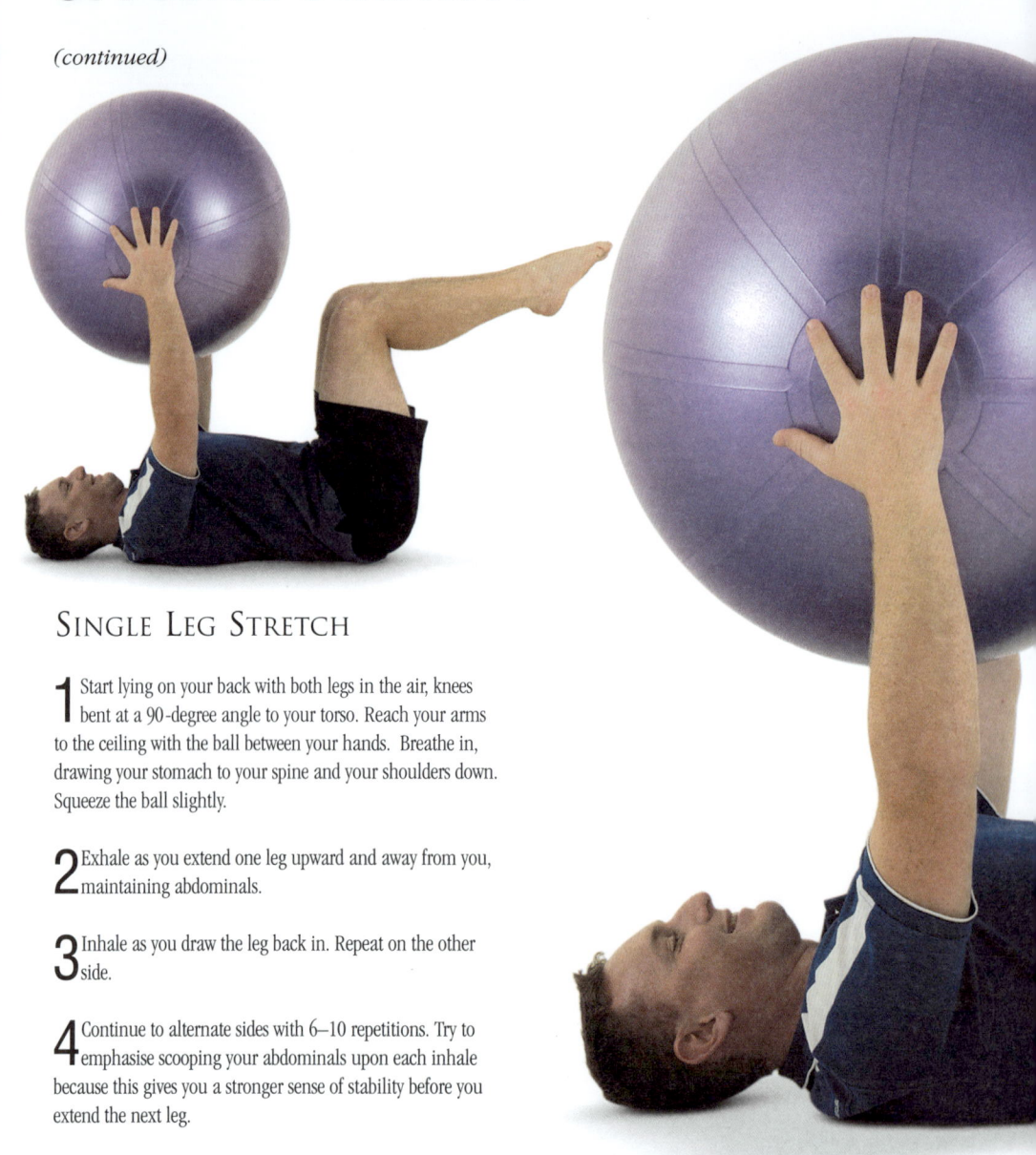

(continued)

Single Leg Stretch

1 Start lying on your back with both legs in the air, knees bent at a 90-degree angle to your torso. Reach your arms to the ceiling with the ball between your hands. Breathe in, drawing your stomach to your spine and your shoulders down. Squeeze the ball slightly.

2 Exhale as you extend one leg upward and away from you, maintaining abdominals.

3 Inhale as you draw the leg back in. Repeat on the other side.

4 Continue to alternate sides with 6–10 repetitions. Try to emphasise scooping your abdominals upon each inhale because this gives you a stronger sense of stability before you extend the next leg.

Progression

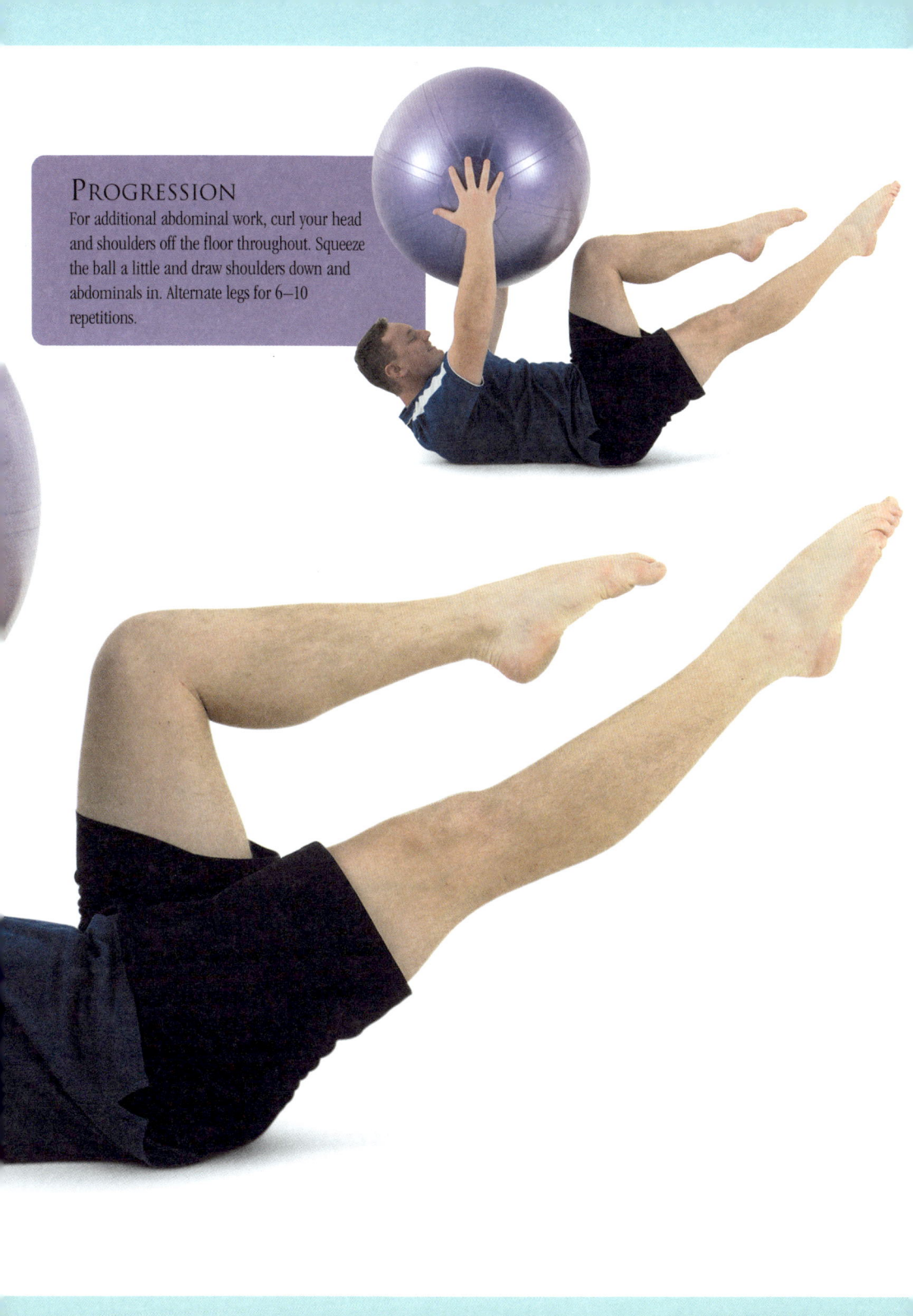

For additional abdominal work, curl your head and shoulders off the floor throughout. Squeeze the ball a little and draw shoulders down and abdominals in. Alternate legs for 6–10 repetitions.

ESSENTIAL BALL • 33

Spinal Mobility & Control

Purpose To promote controlled movement of the spine for strength, segmental coordination and greater mobility.

Side to Side

1 Start with your spine and pelvis in a neutral alignment and the ball directly under your legs, making contact with both your thighs and calves. Once again, your knees are vertically aligned over your hips. Place your arms, palms up, at a moderate distance away from your trunk.

2 Prepare your abdominals and maintain throughout the exercise. Anchor your shoulder blades to the floor so you don't rely on your arms to stabilise you. Inhale as you roll onto one side of your pelvis.

3 Exhale as you return to the centre, ensuring it is your waist muscles that move you. Try not to lead the movement with your legs or back.

4 Alternate sides for 8–10 repetitions.

ESSENTIAL BALL • 35

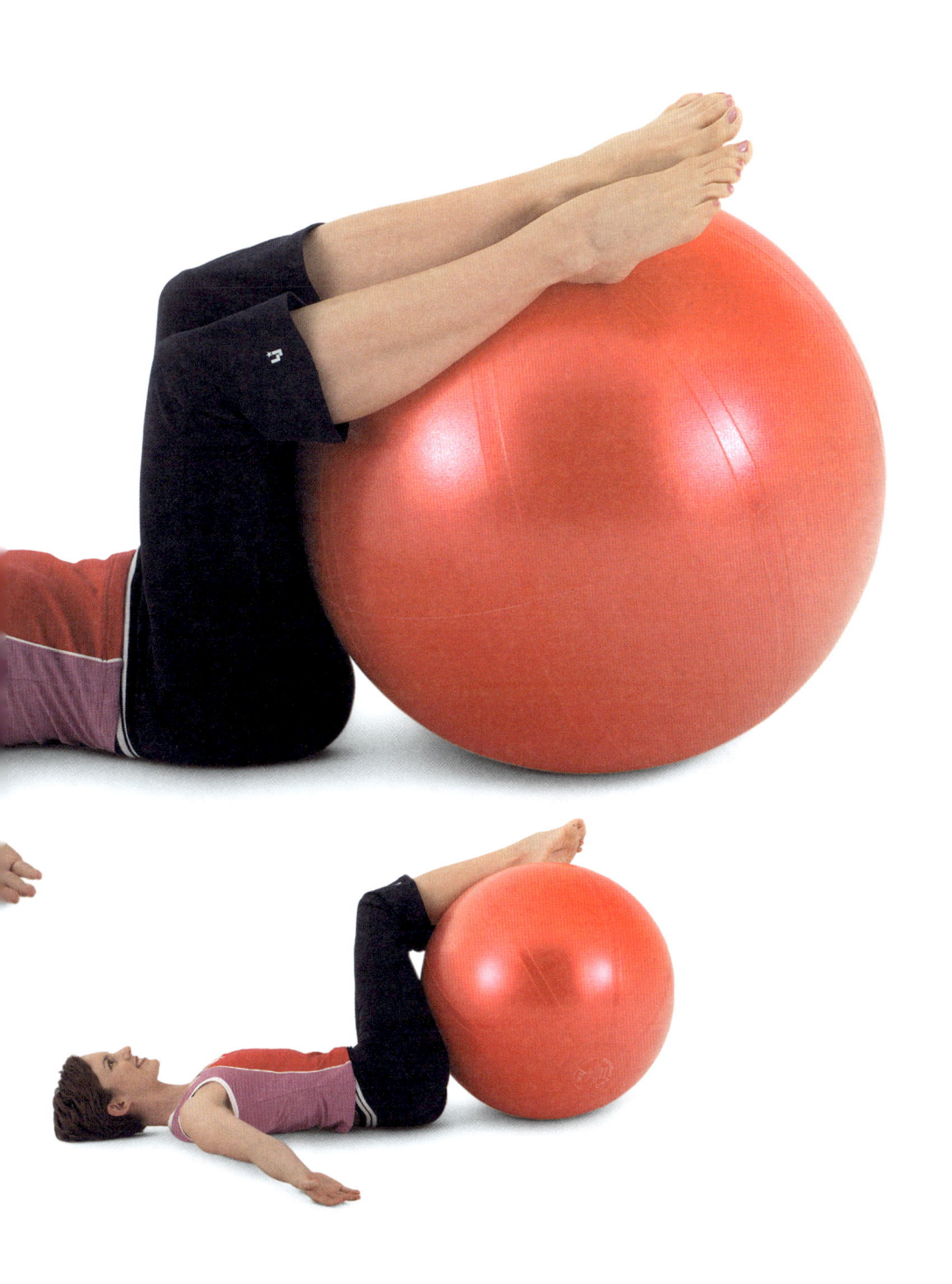

Spinal Mobility & Control

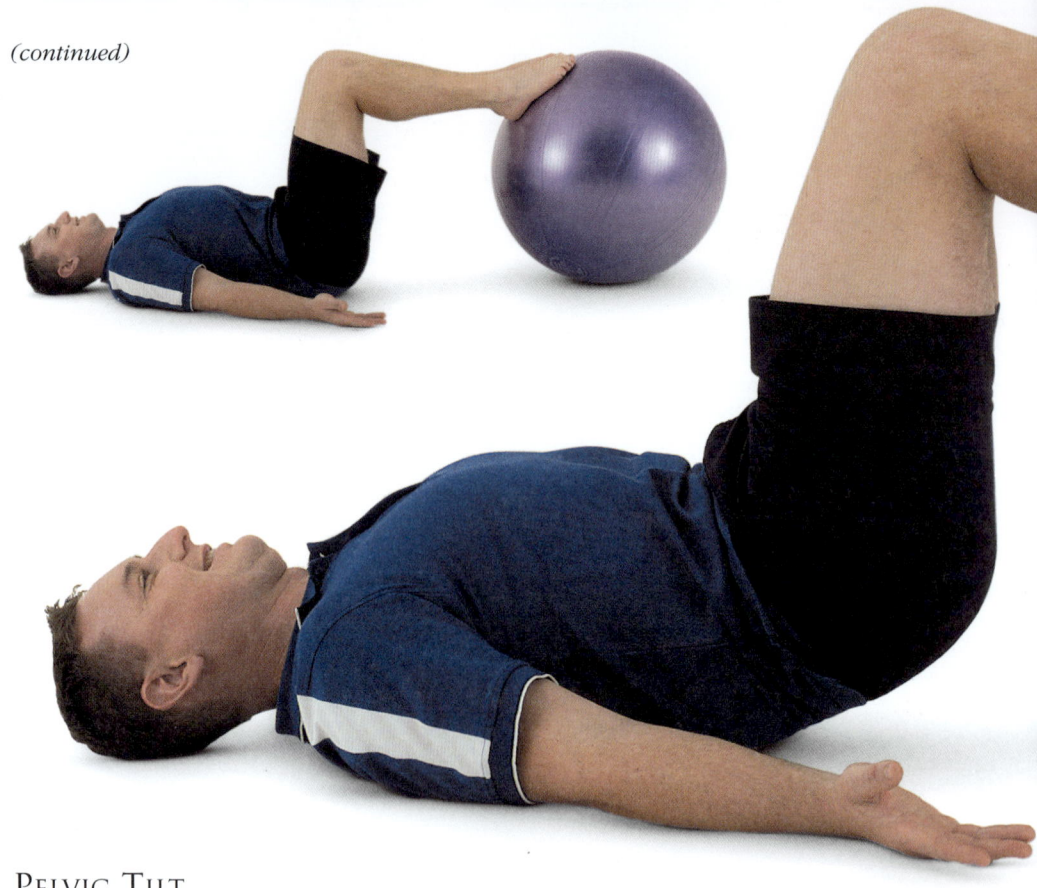

(continued)

Pelvic Tilt

1 Lie on your back with your feet on the ball and your spine and pelvis relaxed in a neutral alignment. Place your arms, palms up, slightly away from your torso, scoop your lower abdominals in and up. Inhale.

2 Exhale as you further draw your abdominals inward to initiate a pelvic tilt backward, stretching your lower back. Ensure that your knees are pointing directly up toward the ceiling and that the backs of your thighs assist with the movement.

3 Inhale laterally, holding the position. Feel the lower part of your gluteals lifting you.

4 Exhale as you roll back to the floor with control, relaxing your hips completely at the end of the roll. Try to keep the ball still throughout and focus purely on mobilising and smoothly articulating your lower back.

5 Repeat 3–4 times.

Progression

For additional legwork and to challenge your stability, try rolling off the floor a little further (exhale) and extending your legs away from you at the top of the movement (inhale). Exhale as you pull the ball back—buttocks high and knees pointing skyward—inhale to hold and maintain. Exhale as you roll and recover. Focus on the lower gluteals and your abdominals. Repeat 3–4 times.

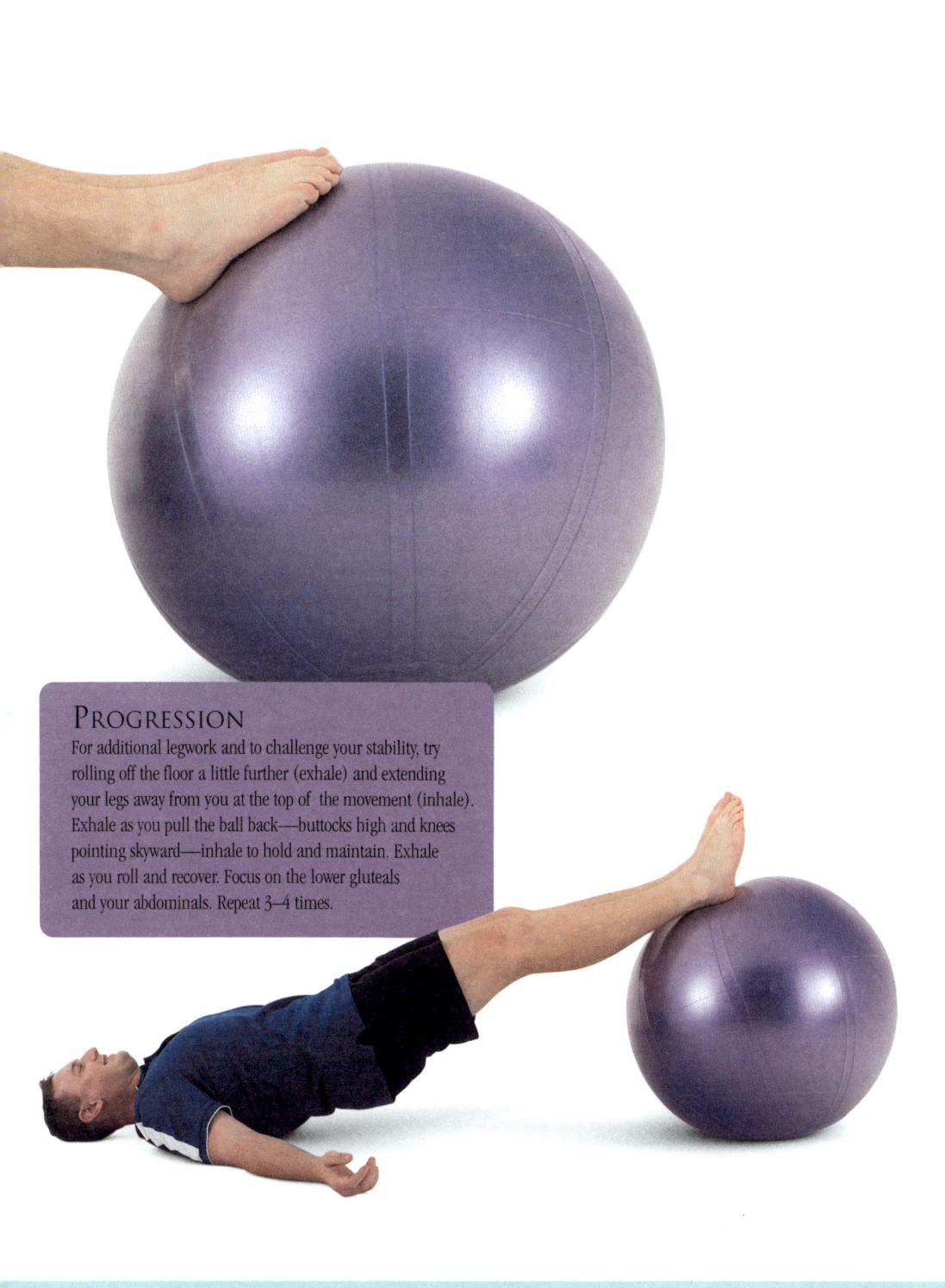

ESSENTIAL BALL • 37

Spinal Mobility & Control

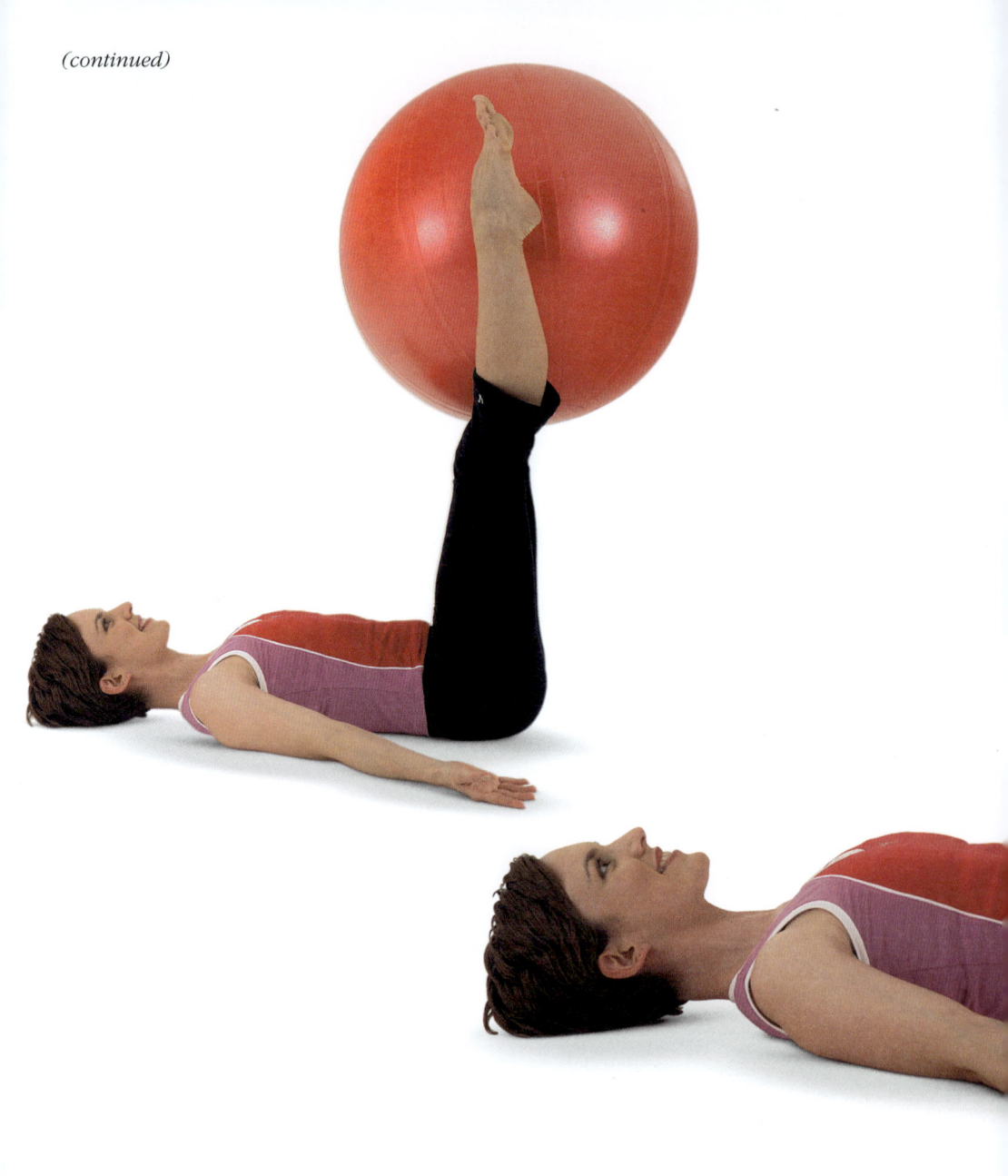

(continued)

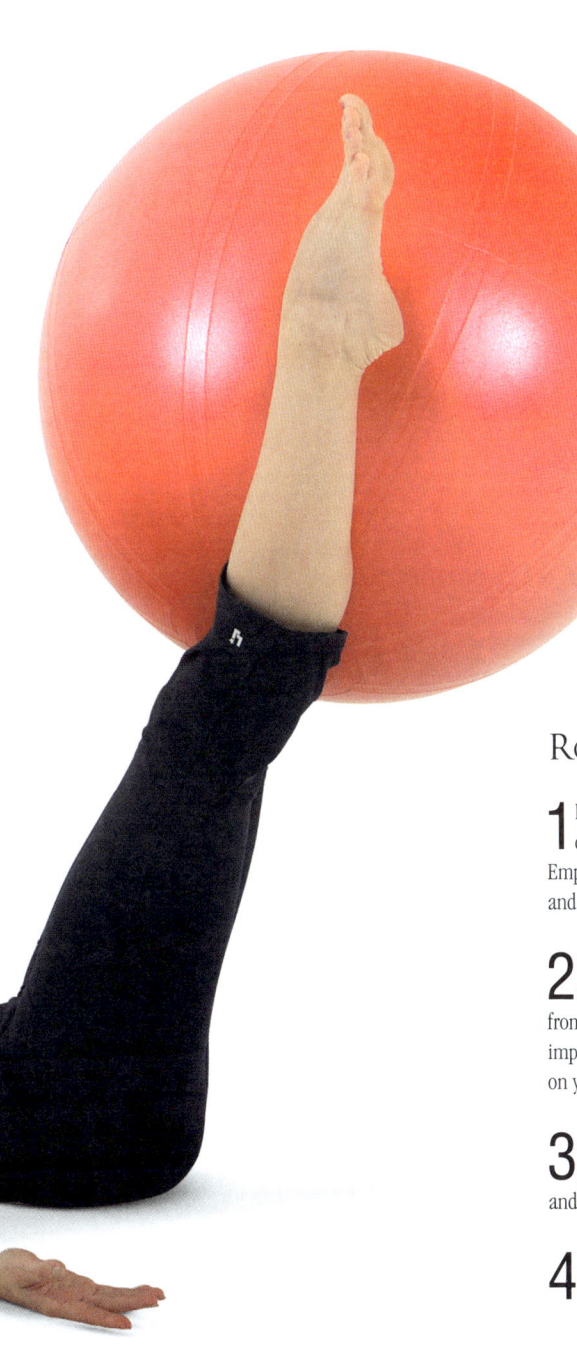

NOTE

Your flexibility and spinal health will determine the suitability of this exercise for you, you may have to bend your knees a little in order to focus on a neutral position of your back and pelvis. Maintain strong abdominals throughout, keep your shoulder blades flat on the floor and your neck relatively tension-free.

ROLLOVER PREP

1 Begin lying on your back with the ball between your calves and ankles. Extend your legs toward the ceiling. Emphasise a Neutral Pelvis, scooping abdominal muscles and tension-free neck.

2 Start with your legs at a 90-degree angle to your body and breathe in as you extend them only very slightly away from you. This is the first movement of a Rollover, where it is important that you develop abdominal control and not rely on your neck, back, legs and arms.

3 As you exhale, draw the legs back towards you. Emphasise your scooping abdominals and squeeze the ball gently and constantly for additional inside thigh work.

4 Repeat 5–6 times.

Spinal Mobility & Control

(continued)

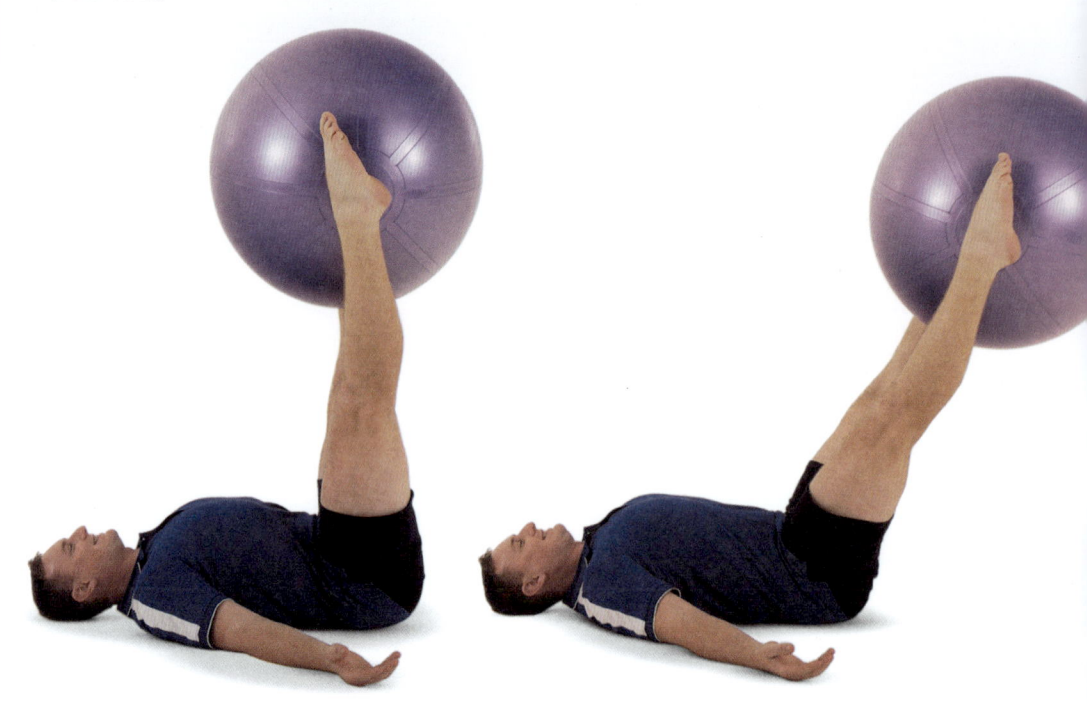

Rollovers

1 Begin as for Rollover Prep. Inhale as you extend your legs slightly away as a preparation for your next manoeuvre.

2 As you exhale, use your abdominals to lift your legs and hips up and over your head. Try to lengthen your waist up toward the ceiling and keep most of your weight on the back of your shoulders instead of compressing your neck.

3 Inhale to maintain your position, legs parallel to the floor—relax in your throat and draw your shoulders down.

4 As you exhale, roll down through your spine with control. Imagine lengthening between each spinal segment.

5 As you return to your neutral alignment, keep your abdominals scooping deeply.

6 Repeat 3–5 times.

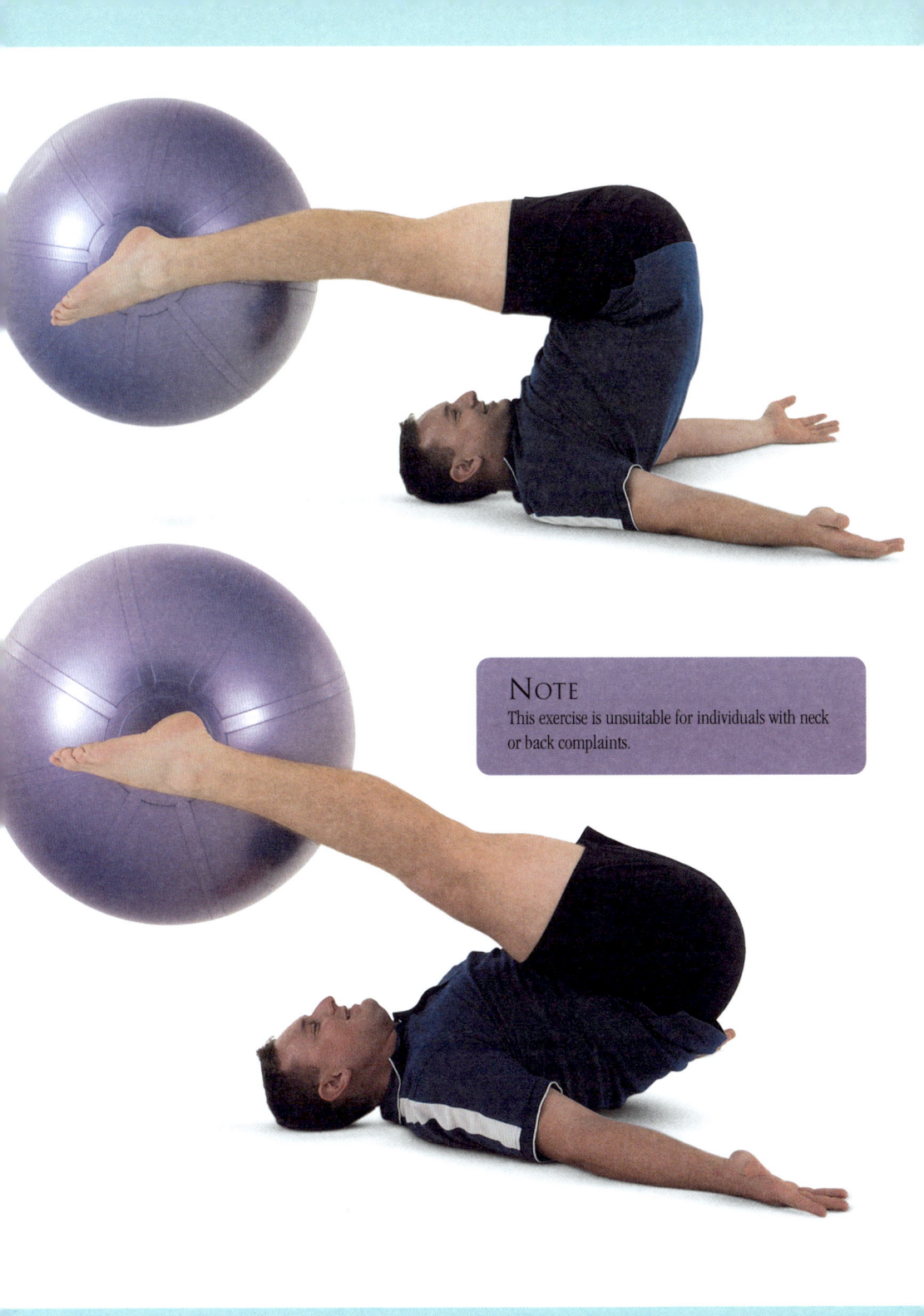

Note
This exercise is unsuitable for individuals with neck or back complaints.

ESSENTIAL BALL • 41

Spinal Rotation

Purpose *To maintain a healthy range of motion throughout the spine and encourage muscular support during twisting movement. Pelvic and shoulder girdle stability are also a component of this exercise.*

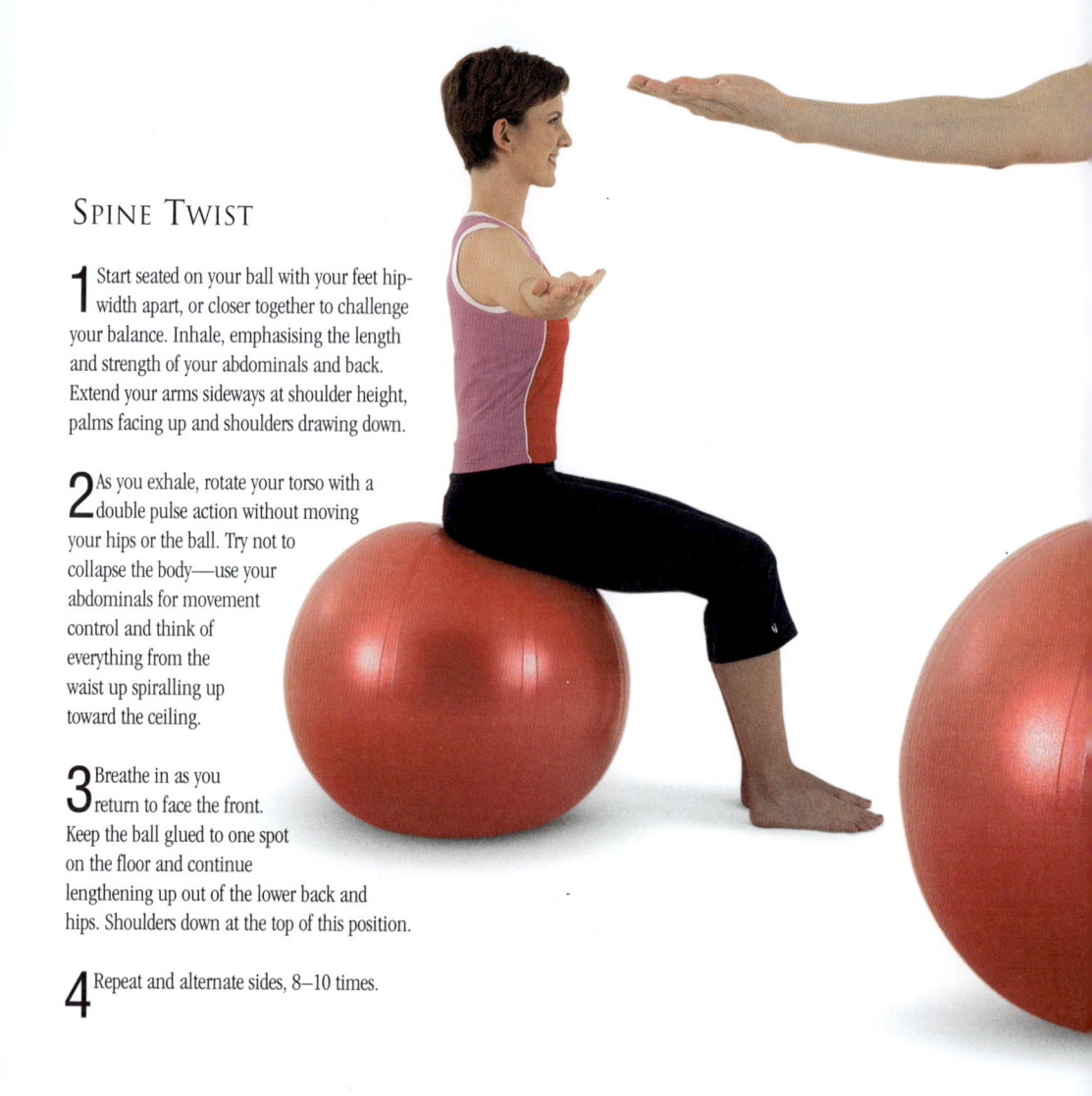

Spine Twist

1 Start seated on your ball with your feet hip-width apart, or closer together to challenge your balance. Inhale, emphasising the length and strength of your abdominals and back. Extend your arms sideways at shoulder height, palms facing up and shoulders drawing down.

2 As you exhale, rotate your torso with a double pulse action without moving your hips or the ball. Try not to collapse the body—use your abdominals for movement control and think of everything from the waist up spiralling up toward the ceiling.

3 Breathe in as you return to face the front. Keep the ball glued to one spot on the floor and continue lengthening up out of the lower back and hips. Shoulders down at the top of this position.

4 Repeat and alternate sides, 8–10 times.

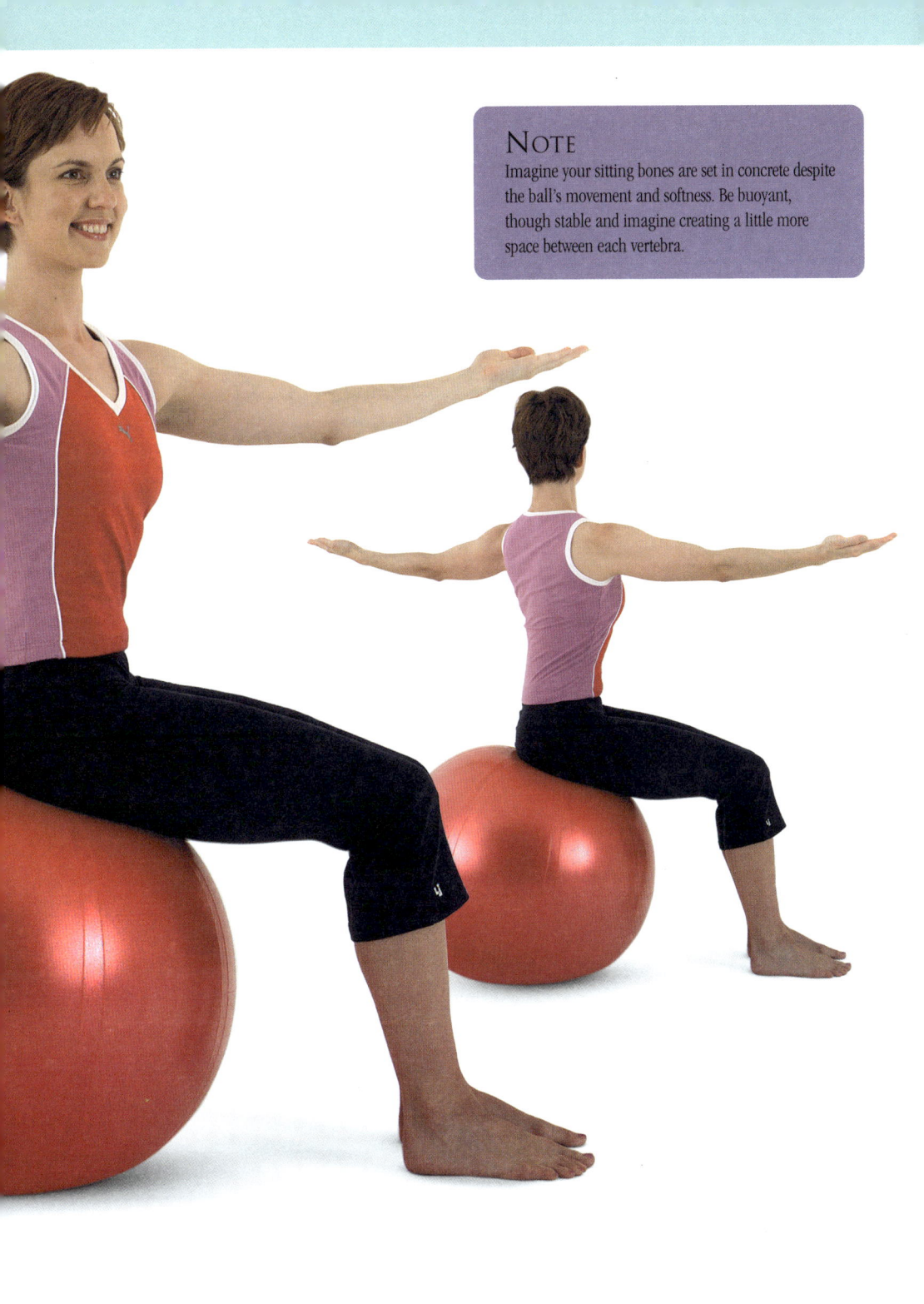

Note

Imagine your sitting bones are set in concrete despite the ball's movement and softness. Be buoyant, though stable and imagine creating a little more space between each vertebra.

Gluteals & Adductors

Purpose *To strengthen and tone the back of the hips and thighs for improved muscle balance. Strong hip, gluteal and inside thigh muscles (adductors) contribute to a stable pelvis and lower back. Abdominal control and core stability are also a strong feature because the ball creates an unstable foundation.*

Bottom Lift Series

1 Prepare by sitting on the ball and walking forward so that you roll your pelvis under and lie on the ball. Continue walking until your head, neck and shoulders are fully supported and place your hands either under your head or on your hips. Ensure that your knee alignment is correct, with your kneecaps pointing forward and your knees not too far out over your toes. Heels should almost touch each other and toes should be slightly splayed.

2 Your focus should now remain on the muscles at the tops of the back of your thighs and the lower section of your buttocks (hamstrings and gluteals). Try to maintain a long sensation of your waist and thighs. Inhale as you lower your pelvis, without moving the ball.

3 Exhale, lift your pelvis using your hamstrings and gluteals without over-using your lower back. Think of stretching the fronts of your thighs upward and long.

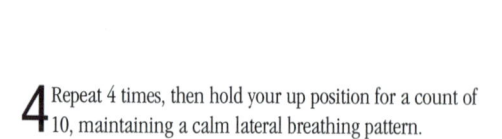

4 Repeat 4 times, then hold your up position for a count of 10, maintaining a calm lateral breathing pattern.

5 After sustaining your Bottom Lift, proceed to squeeze the tops of your thighs together with small, quick pulses. Inhale for 4 pulses, exhale for 4 pulses. Repeat this breathing sequence as you continue to squeeze, 5–6 times. Maintain focus on the muscles of the lower part of your buttocks throughout.

ESSENTIAL BALL • 45

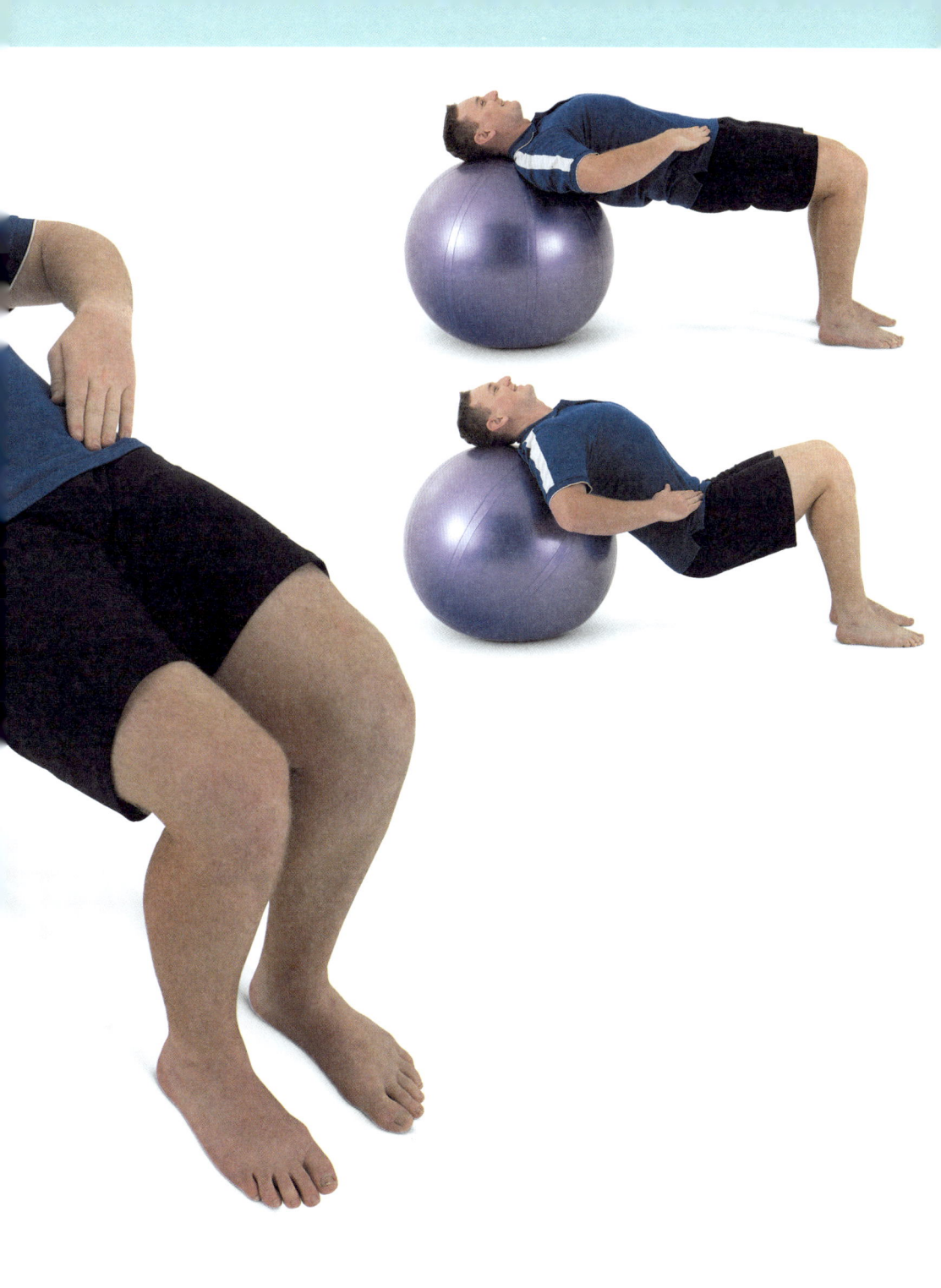

Gluteals & Adductors

(continued)

Side Balance

1 Lie on your side with the ball between your ankles. Keep the legs slightly forward of your hips and lie directly on your side so that you can balance on your thighbone. Lengthen your legs away from you and focus on your abdominals—especially your underneath side, as that is what helps you gain balance.

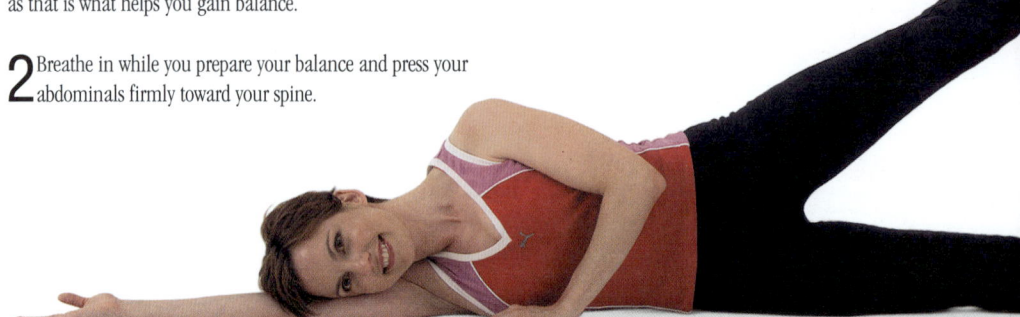

2 Breathe in while you prepare your balance and press your abdominals firmly toward your spine.

3 As you exhale, squeeze your top leg into the ball and lengthen your waist.

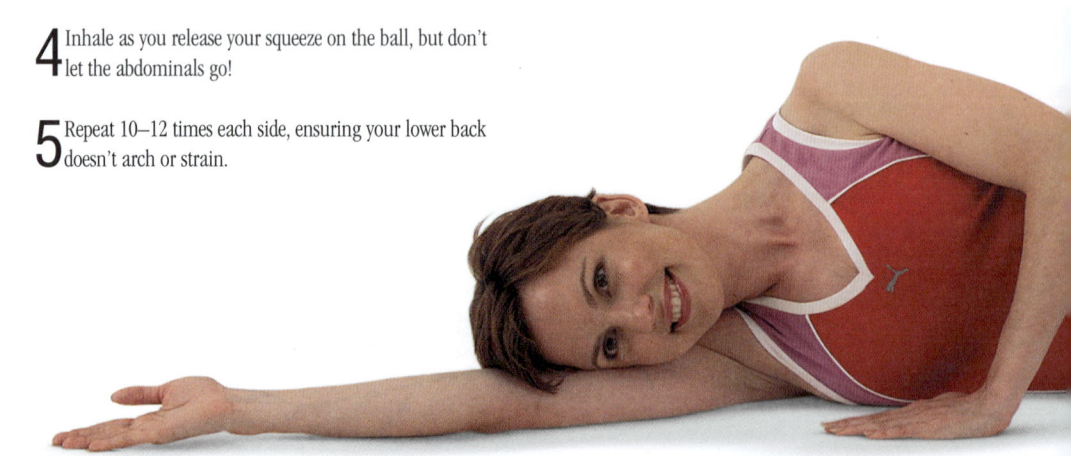

4 Inhale as you release your squeeze on the ball, but don't let the abdominals go!

5 Repeat 10–12 times each side, ensuring your lower back doesn't arch or strain.

Progression

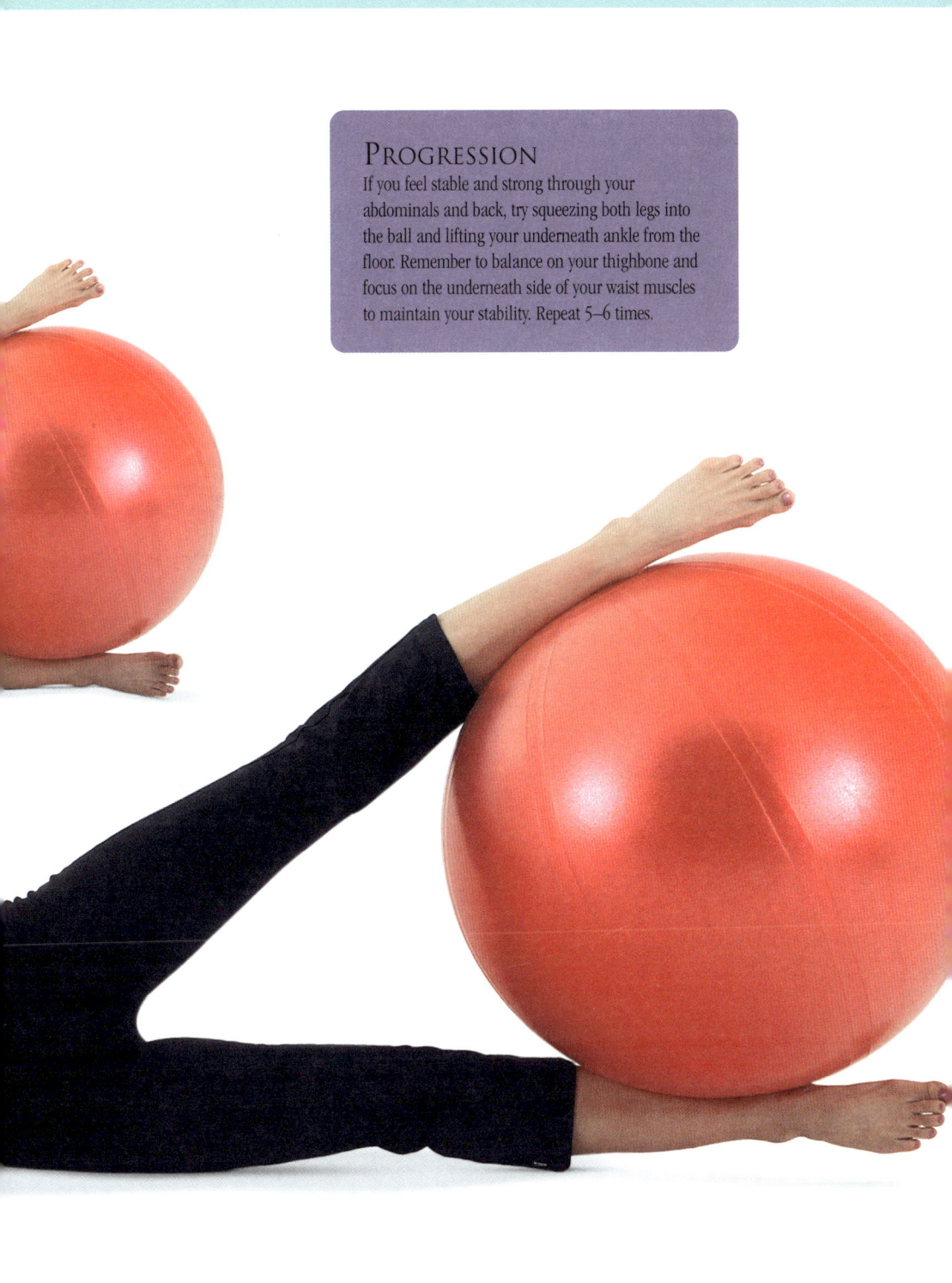

If you feel stable and strong through your abdominals and back, try squeezing both legs into the ball and lifting your underneath ankle from the floor. Remember to balance on your thighbone and focus on the underneath side of your waist muscles to maintain your stability. Repeat 5–6 times.

Scapula Stability & Back Strengthening

Purpose *To develop and strengthen the muscles of the middle and upper back for better posture. Increasing the endurance of these postural muscles will help alleviate neck and shoulder tension.*

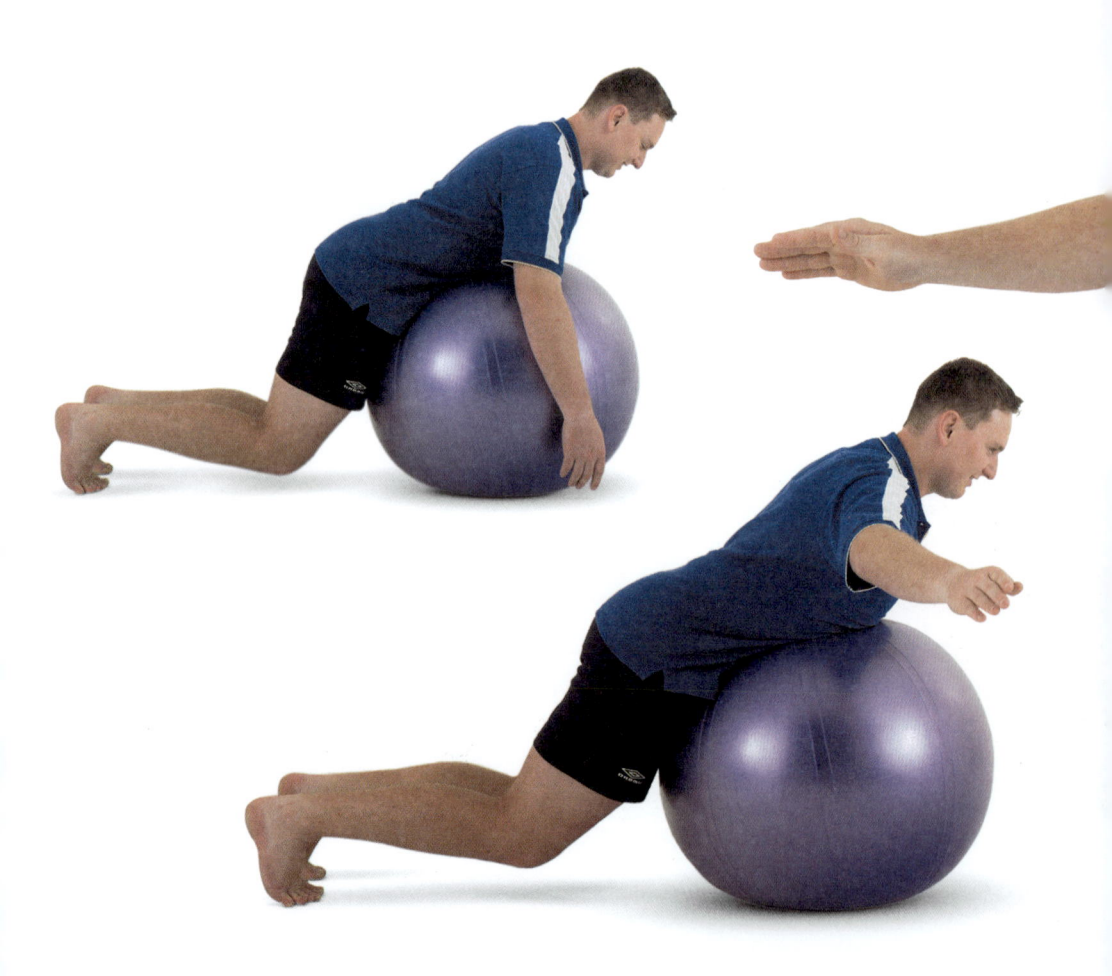

Arm Openings

1 Begin kneeling with the ball in front of you and against your thighs. Roll forward on the ball so your knees lift just off the floor and push the lower part of your ribcage gently into the ball so you can lift your chest bone slightly —this action will allow you better use of the postural muscles of your upper back, relieving stress from your neck. Keep your abdominals lifted and your shoulder blades drawing down flat against your ribcage throughout. Inhale to prepare.

2 As you exhale, raise your arms sideways without hitching your shoulders up or squeezing your shoulder blades. The idea of scapula stability is to move your shoulder joints without allowing your shoulder blades to move from their ideal anatomical alignment. Hold momentarily.

3 Lower your arms as you inhale.

4 Repeat 6–10 times.

Progression
Add hand weights of a kilo or half a kilo to challenge the stability of your back and shoulder girdle and gain further strength. The weight should not be so heavy that muscle strain occurs in the neck. Focus on the middle of your back bracing and keeping your abdominals lifted.

Scapula Stability & Back Strengthening

(continued)

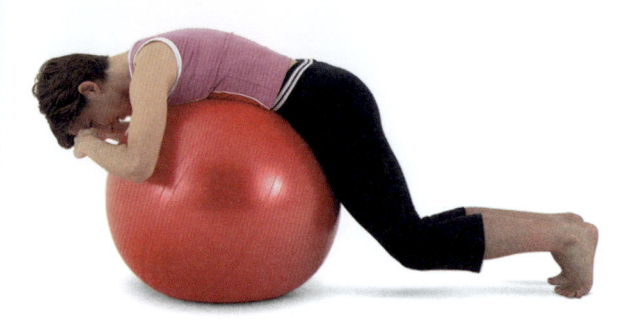

Back Extension

1 Begin as for Arm Openings, though place your fingers under your forehead and drape yourself forward over the ball. Engage your abdominals and prepare yourself to keep the front of your torso stable against the ball.

2 Breathe in as you lift your upper torso—imagine bending from your mid-thoracic area. Ensure your abdominals remain lifted and your shoulders draw down.

3 Exhale as your lower yourself. Maintain the lift of your abdominals so that you're prepared and stable for the next repetition.

4 Repeat 6–10 times.

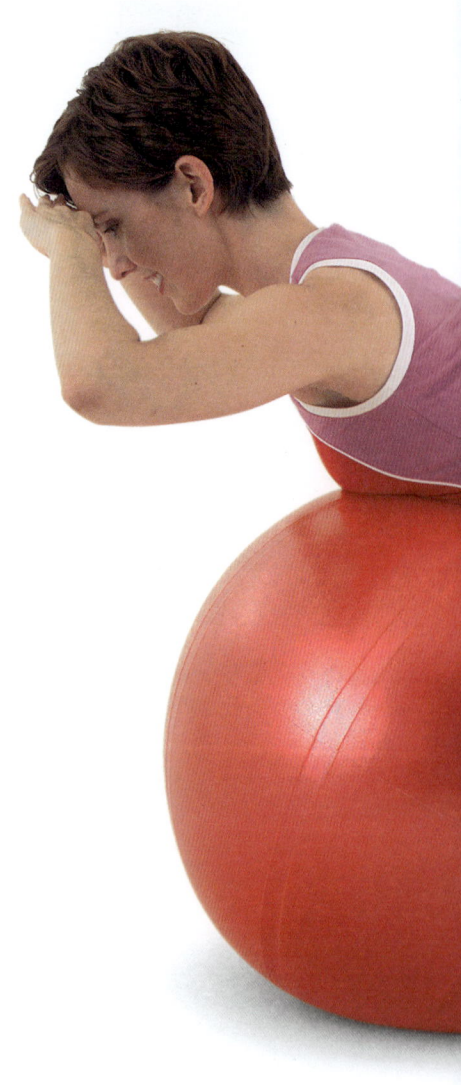

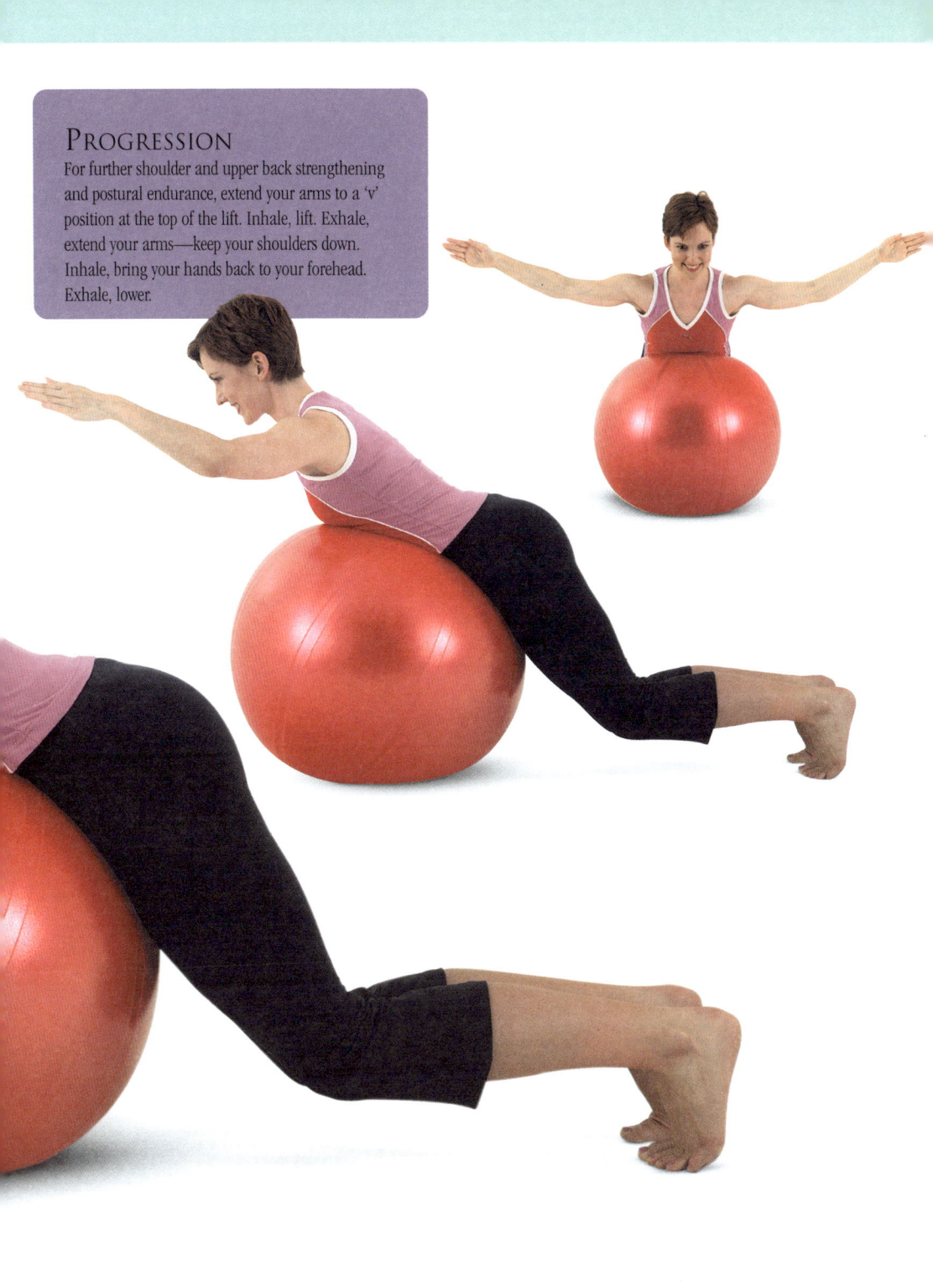

Progression

For further shoulder and upper back strengthening and postural endurance, extend your arms to a 'v' position at the top of the lift. Inhale, lift. Exhale, extend your arms—keep your shoulders down. Inhale, bring your hands back to your forehead. Exhale, lower.

ESSENTIAL BALL • 51

FULL BODY INTEGRATION

Purpose To ultimately challenge the individual's ability to have a true 'full body' focus, combining the need to stabilise the lower back with strong abdominal muscles, maintain a steady shoulder girdle position and to coordinate isolated movement of the limbs.

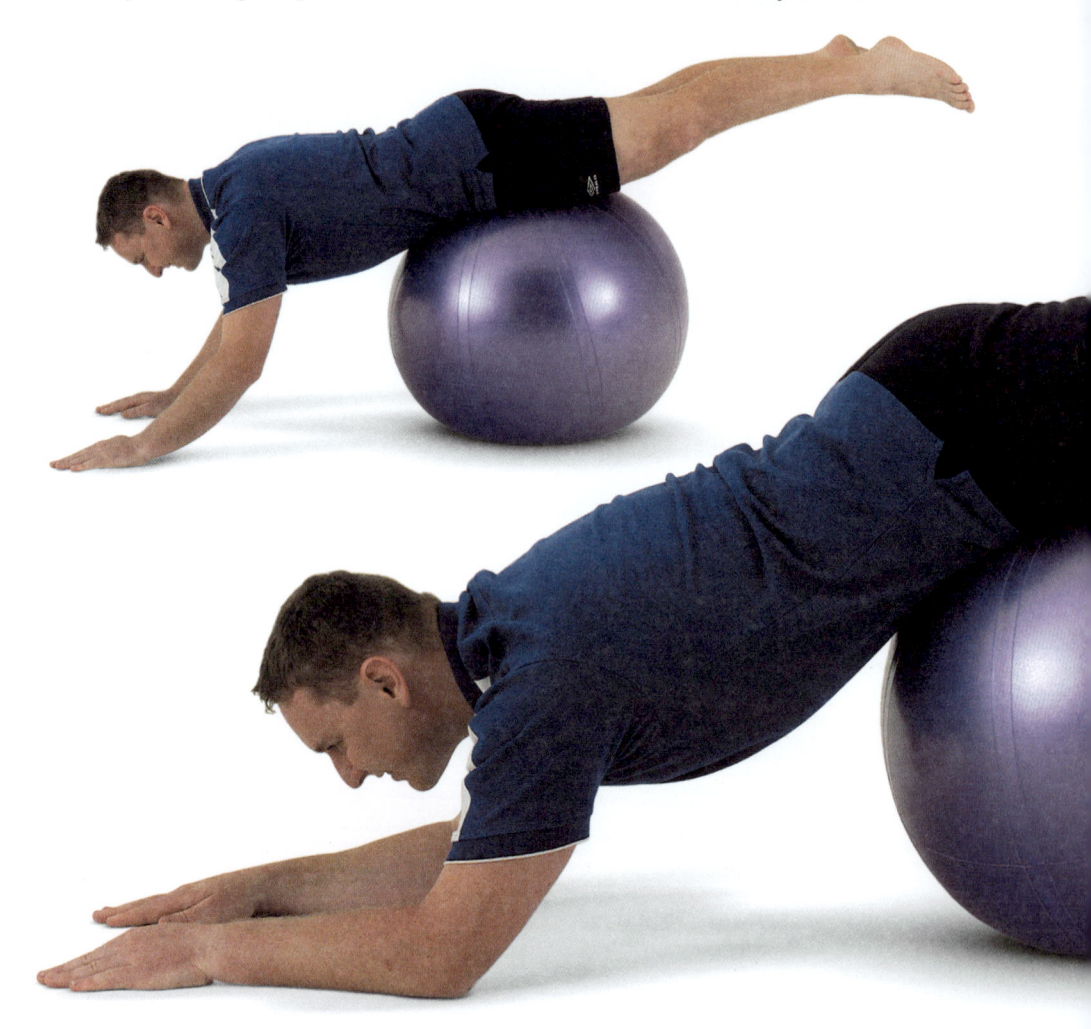

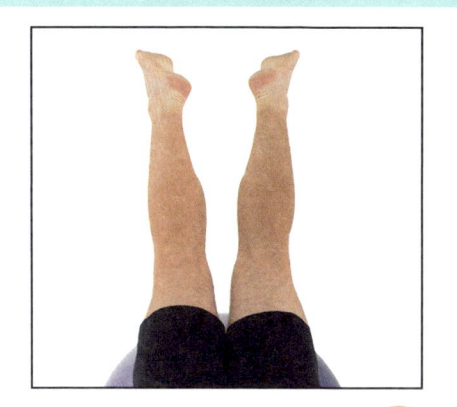

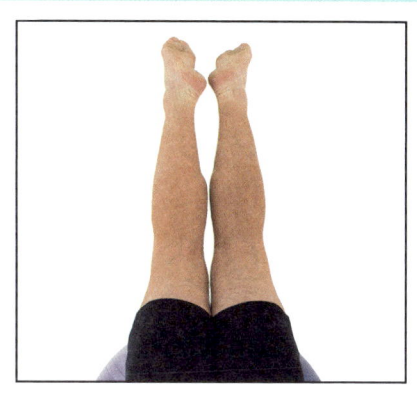

Leg Beats

1 Begin kneeling with the ball in front of you and roll forward so that your thighs and pelvis are on the ball. Support your weight by your hands or elbows and keep your shoulder blades flat against your ribs with your abdominals lifting, acting like a 'sling' to support your lower back. This upper body position must remain stable throughout.

2 Now, focus on a long waist and strong long legs. You may slightly turn your thighs out. Beat your legs together with small crisp sideways movements, from the tops of the back of your thighs, down to your heels. Inhale for 4 beats, exhale for 4 beats.

3 Repeat 6–10 times.

Note
If you are on your hands slightly soften your elbow joints so that they point backwards and keep your shoulders directly over your hands. Emphasise abdominals up, nose down and shoulder blades down and flat.

Full Body Integration

(continued)

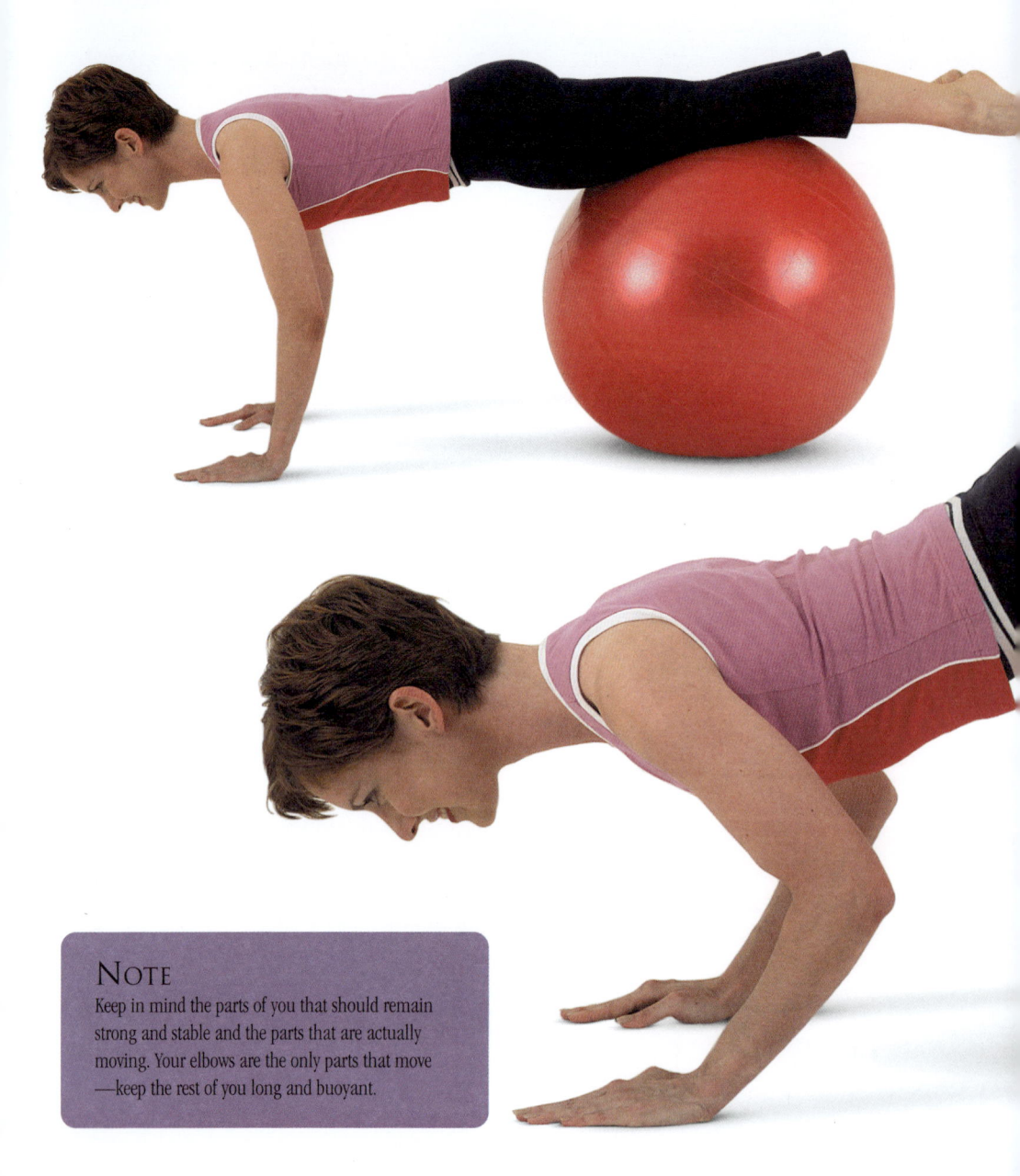

> **Note**
> Keep in mind the parts of you that should remain strong and stable and the parts that are actually moving. Your elbows are the only parts that move —keep the rest of you long and buoyant.

ESSENTIAL BALL • 54

Push-ups

1 Begin as for Leg Beats and walk forward only as far as you are able to maintain a stable back and shoulder girdle. Start with the ball under your thighs and walk your hands further away from the ball as you are able to progress your position. Hands under shoulders, shoulder blades flat, abdominals lifted and waist and thighs 'long'.

2 Inhale as you bend your elbows so they point backward. Shoulder blades should not squeeze together and lower back should not sag. Remember—nose down, abdominals up.

3 Exhale as you press up, pushing through the heels of your hands.

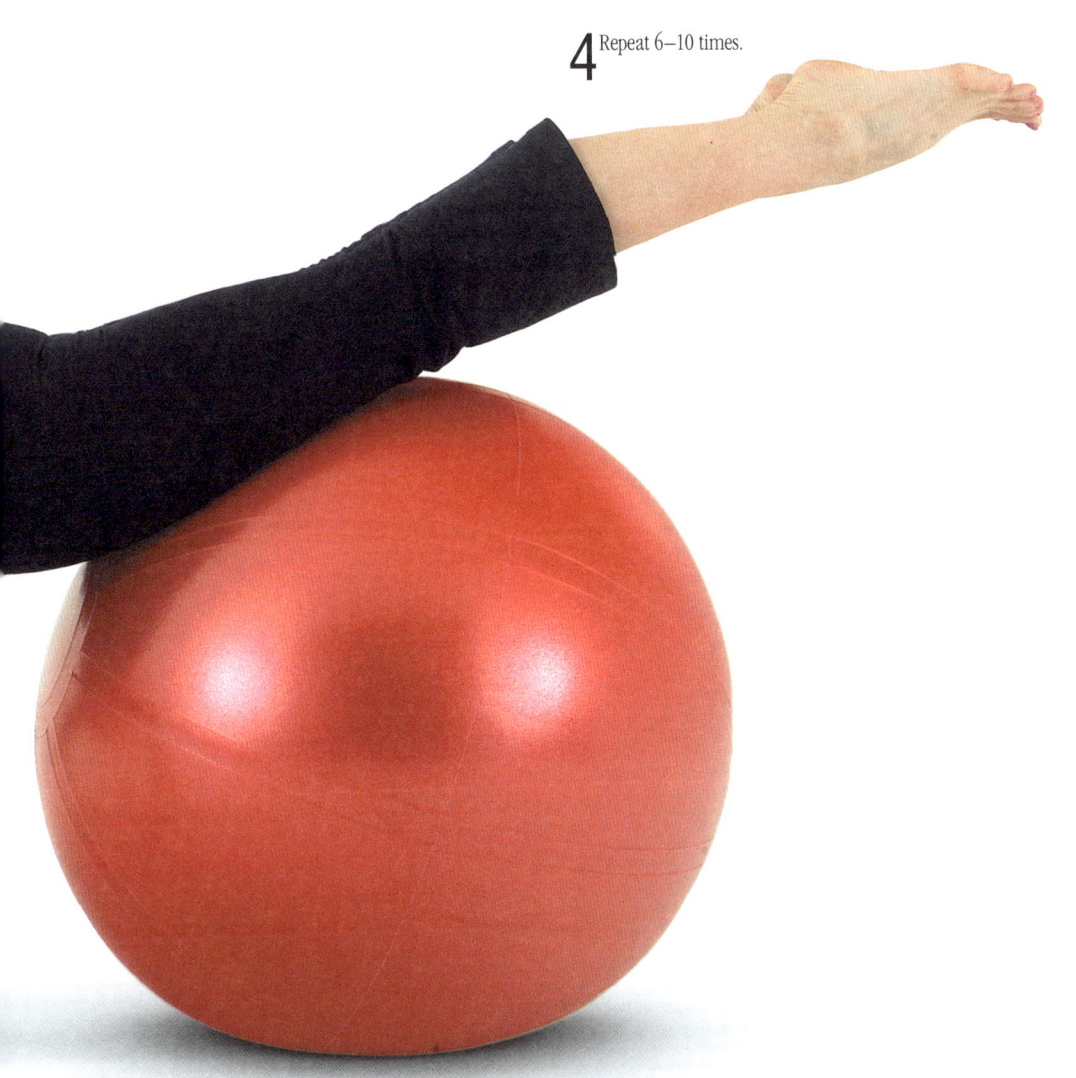

4 Repeat 6–10 times.

STRETCH & RELAX

Purpose *To release muscle and joint tension and achieve more suppleness and mobility. After exercising muscles it is beneficial to stretch them so that they maintain or gain length and are less susceptible to strain or injury. After stretching, your mind and body feel invigorated.*

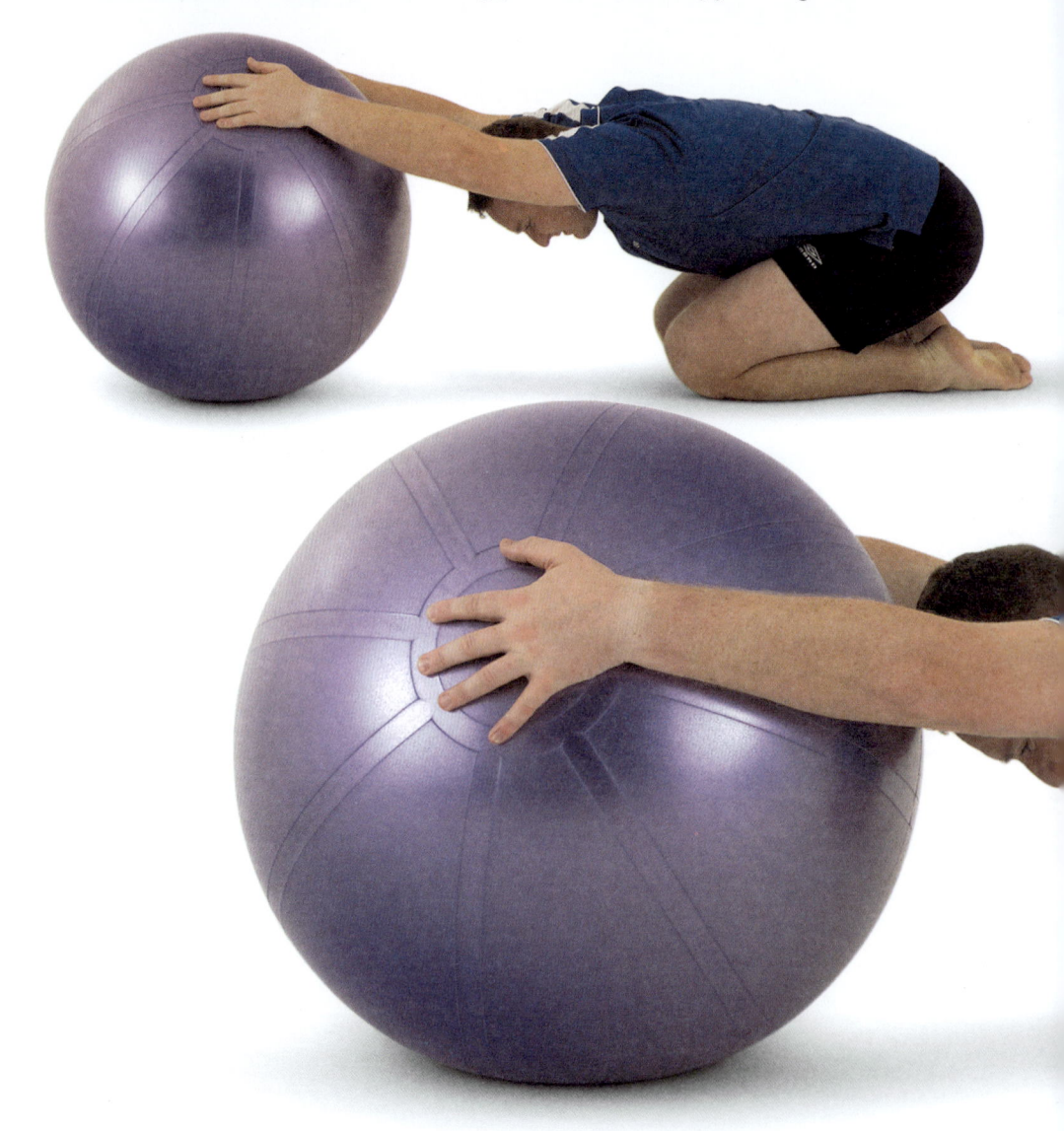

Thoracic Push Through

1 Kneel with the ball in front of you and place both hands on top of the ball. Allow the ball to roll away so that your hips are directly over your knees. If this is too precarious simply sit on your feet.

2 Allow your chest to fall through your arms toward the floor. Take care with your shoulders—you may have to bend or straighten your elbows to adjust your position more comfortably. The idea is to gently mobilise and release your mid-thoracic spine, where a lot of postural tension builds up.

3 Breathe normally and relax for 5–6 full breaths. Repeat if necessary.

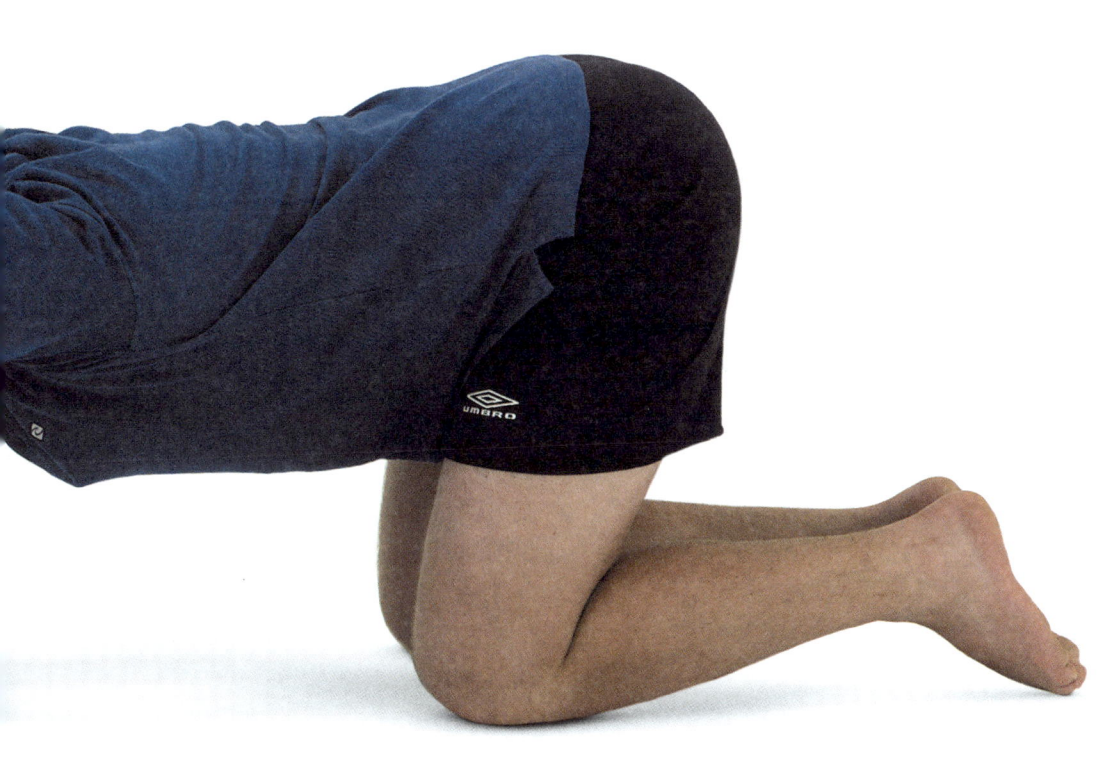

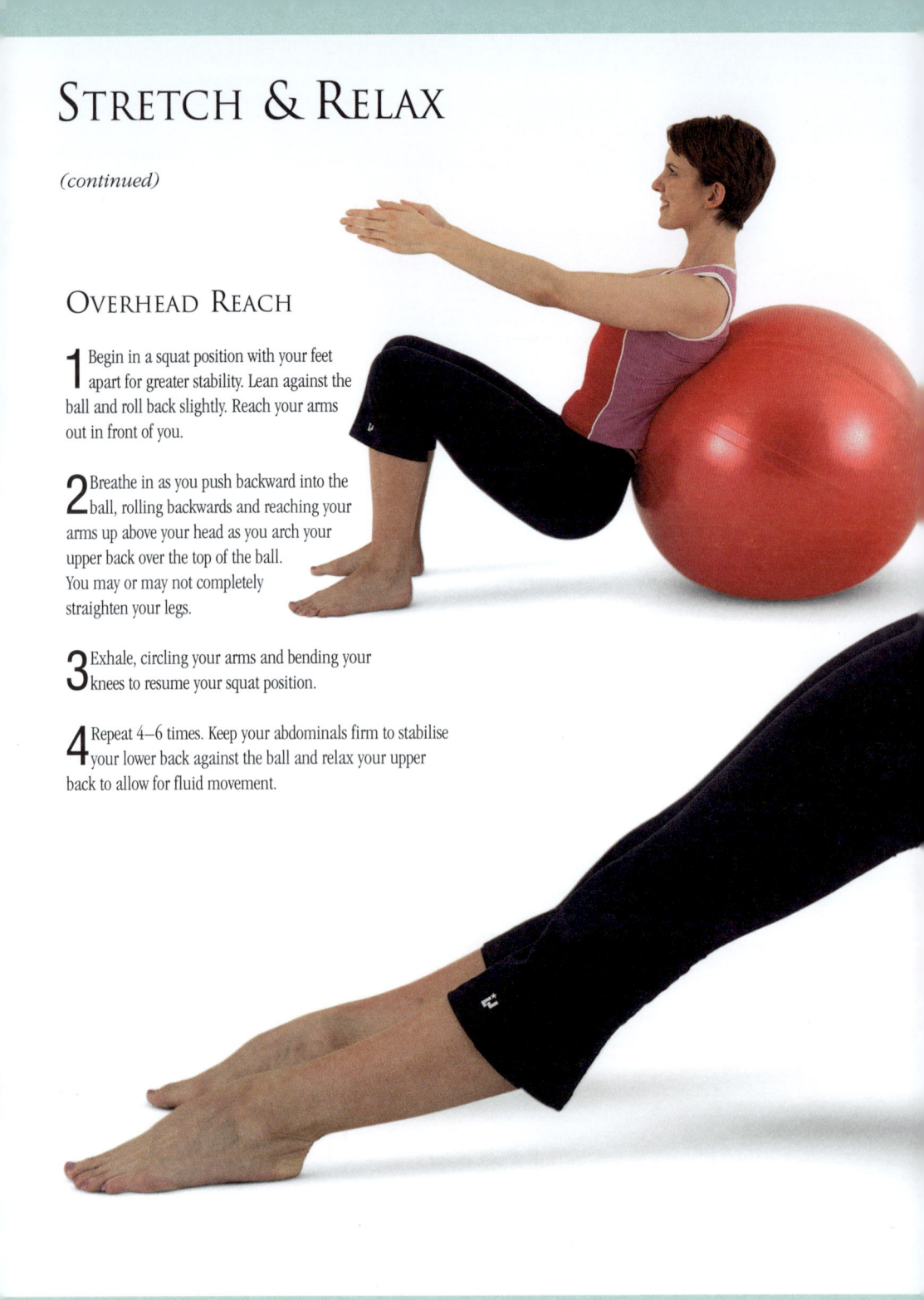

Stretch & Relax

(continued)

Overhead Reach

1 Begin in a squat position with your feet apart for greater stability. Lean against the ball and roll back slightly. Reach your arms out in front of you.

2 Breathe in as you push backward into the ball, rolling backwards and reaching your arms up above your head as you arch your upper back over the top of the ball. You may or may not completely straighten your legs.

3 Exhale, circling your arms and bending your knees to resume your squat position.

4 Repeat 4–6 times. Keep your abdominals firm to stabilise your lower back against the ball and relax your upper back to allow for fluid movement.

Note

Upon returning from the back extension, 'chin to chest' first before continuing to bend your knees. If you require neck support, place your hands behind your head and neck and perhaps not extend quite as far backwards.

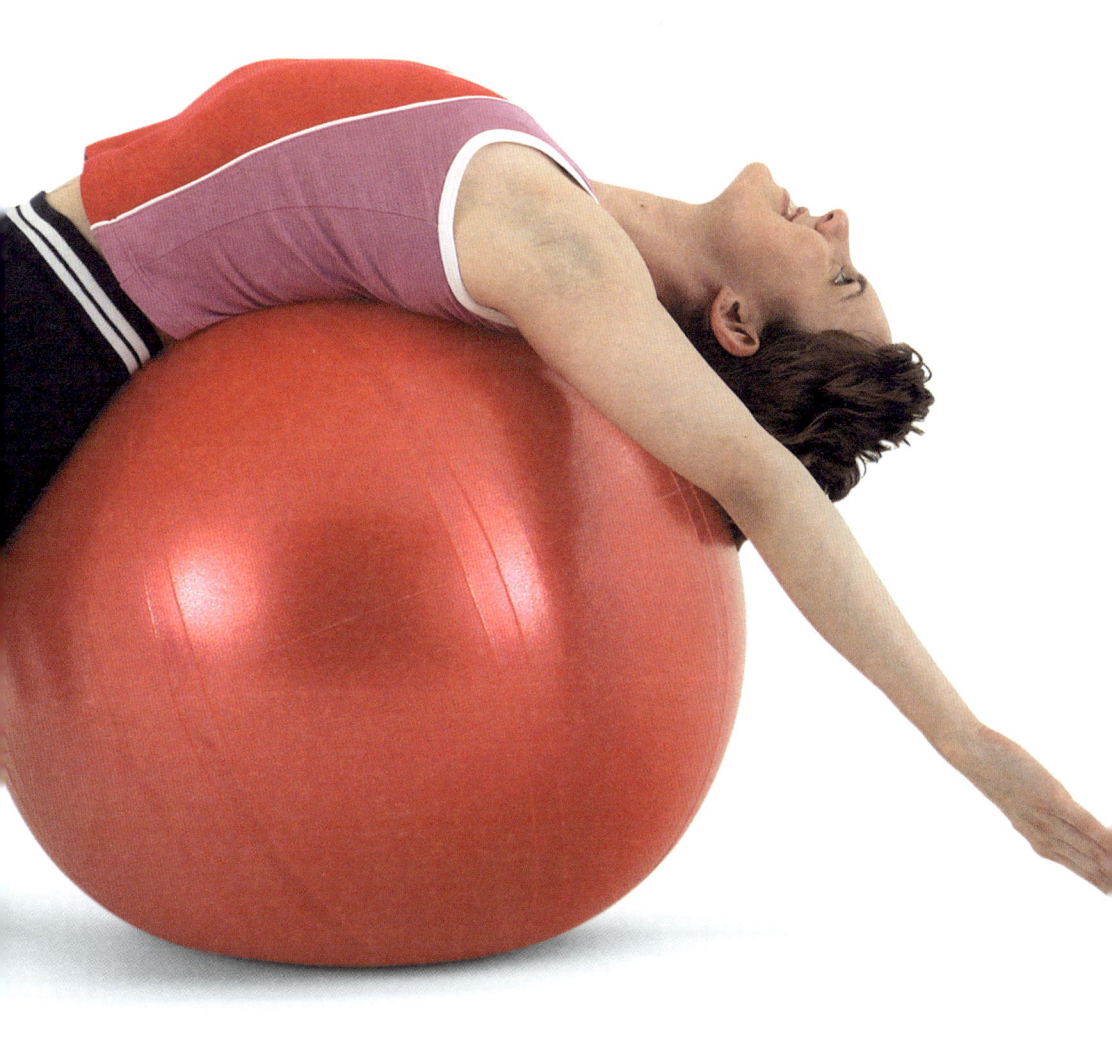

Stretch & Relax

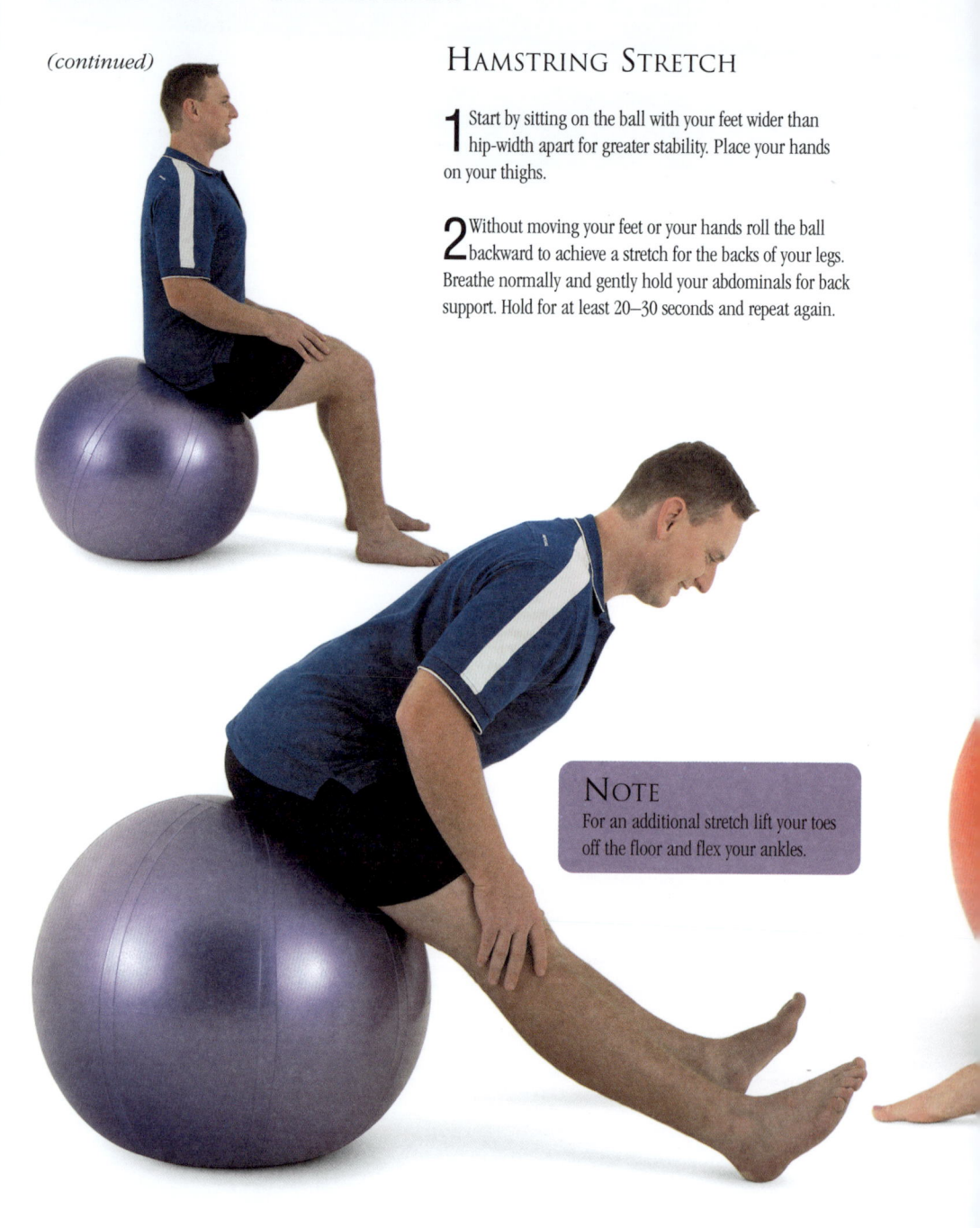

(continued)

Hamstring Stretch

1 Start by sitting on the ball with your feet wider than hip-width apart for greater stability. Place your hands on your thighs.

2 Without moving your feet or your hands roll the ball backward to achieve a stretch for the backs of your legs. Breathe normally and gently hold your abdominals for back support. Hold for at least 20–30 seconds and repeat again.

Note
For an additional stretch lift your toes off the floor and flex your ankles.

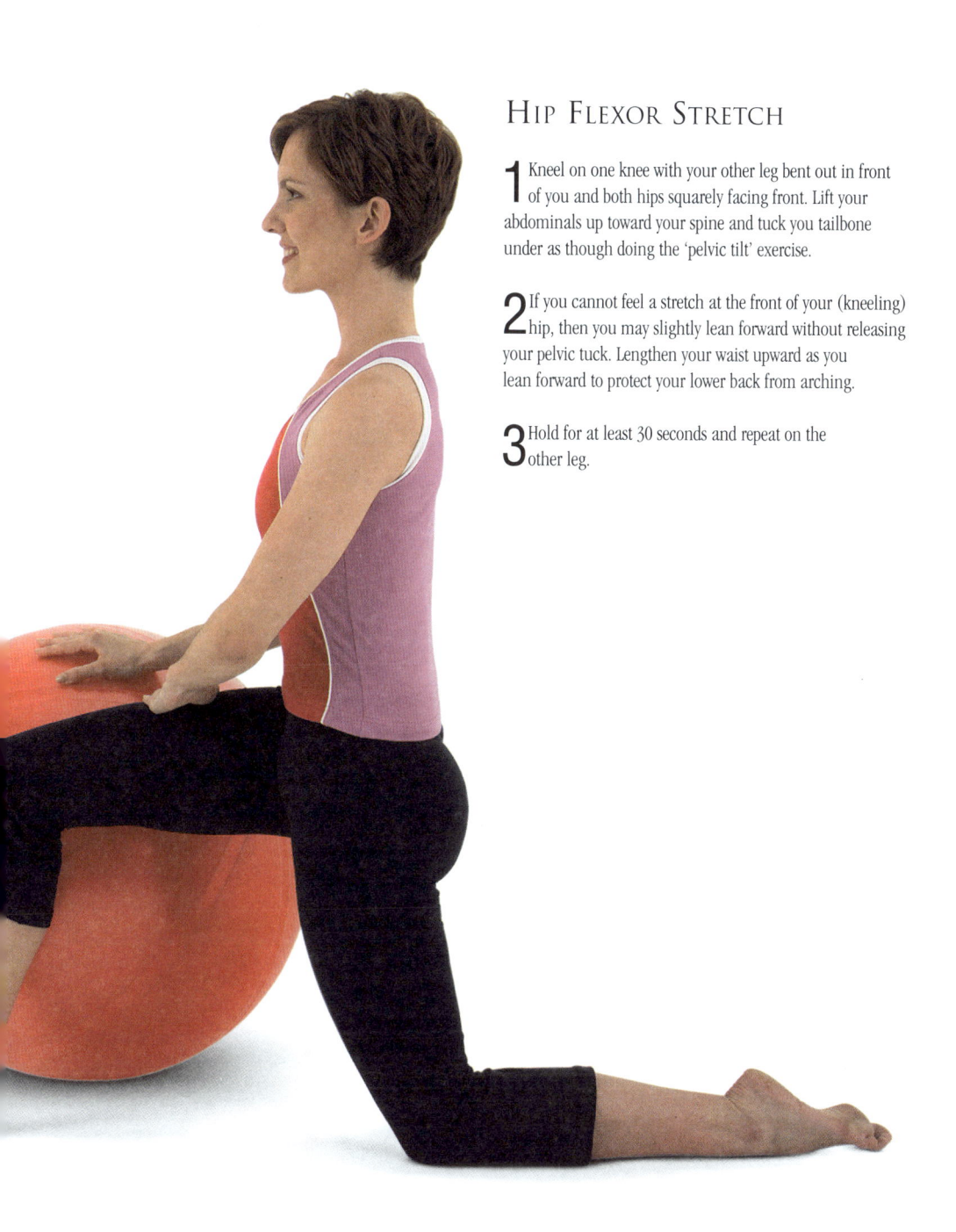

Hip Flexor Stretch

1 Kneel on one knee with your other leg bent out in front of you and both hips squarely facing front. Lift your abdominals up toward your spine and tuck you tailbone under as though doing the 'pelvic tilt' exercise.

2 If you cannot feel a stretch at the front of your (kneeling) hip, then you may slightly lean forward without releasing your pelvic tuck. Lengthen your waist upward as you lean forward to protect your lower back from arching.

3 Hold for at least 30 seconds and repeat on the other leg.

Glossary

Adductors
Muscles of the inner thighs, which draw the legs together.

Gluteals
Muscle group of the buttocks, which contribute to hip movement and stability of the pelvis and lumbar spine.

Hamstrings
Muscle group of the back of the thigh, from the sitting bone to the back of the knee, which bends the knee or assists in backward leg motion.

Hip Flexors
Muscles at the front of the hip that lift the thigh toward the torso.

Oblique Abdominals
Muscles at the sides of the abdomen that predominantly twist, or rotate, the torso.

Scapula
The shoulder blade, which makes up part of the shoulder joint.

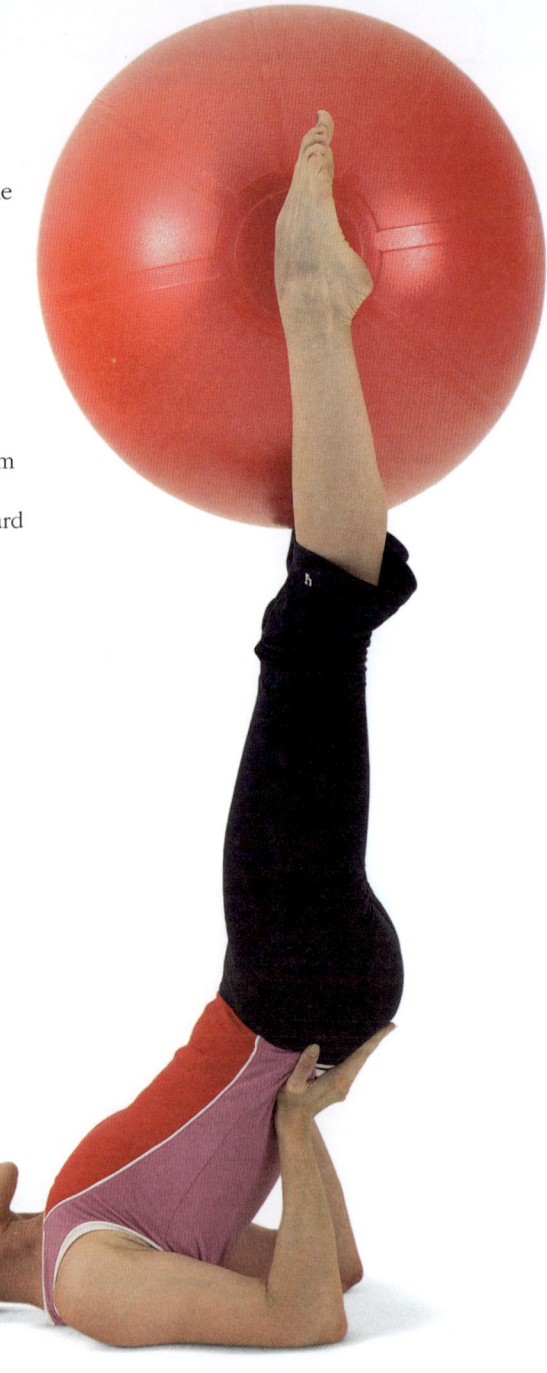

CONCLUSION

Pilates is a unique movement re-education system because it acknowledges the body as the integrated whole that it is, and aims for each individual to develop to their fitness potential.

The Pilates way of moving is a superior method of training muscles for greater endurance, both for postural benefit and dynamically. Core strengthening is becoming more widely practised and Pilates techniques have long been renowned for including this fundamental component in overall fitness training. In essence, the Pilates Method is built upon intuitive movement pathways.

This practice encourages optimal full-range movement of all joints, as well as improving the grace and efficiency with which the body moves.

The beauty of practising Pilates is that improvements in strength, stability and freer moving joints are achieved by persevering with a methodical and frequent approach to the work. Each time you begin your workout remember to apply yourself mentally—think logically about what you are doing, breathe in a regular manner and purposefully move your body. Be kind to your body and condition it with care—it has to last you a lifetime!

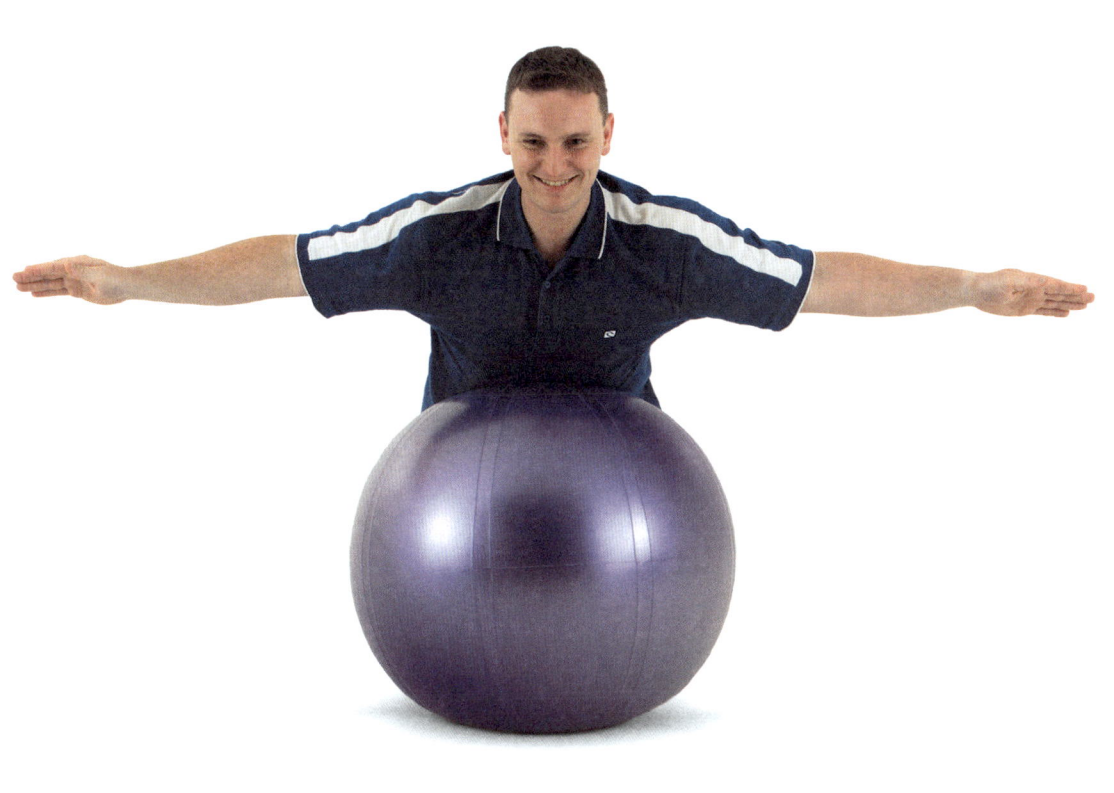

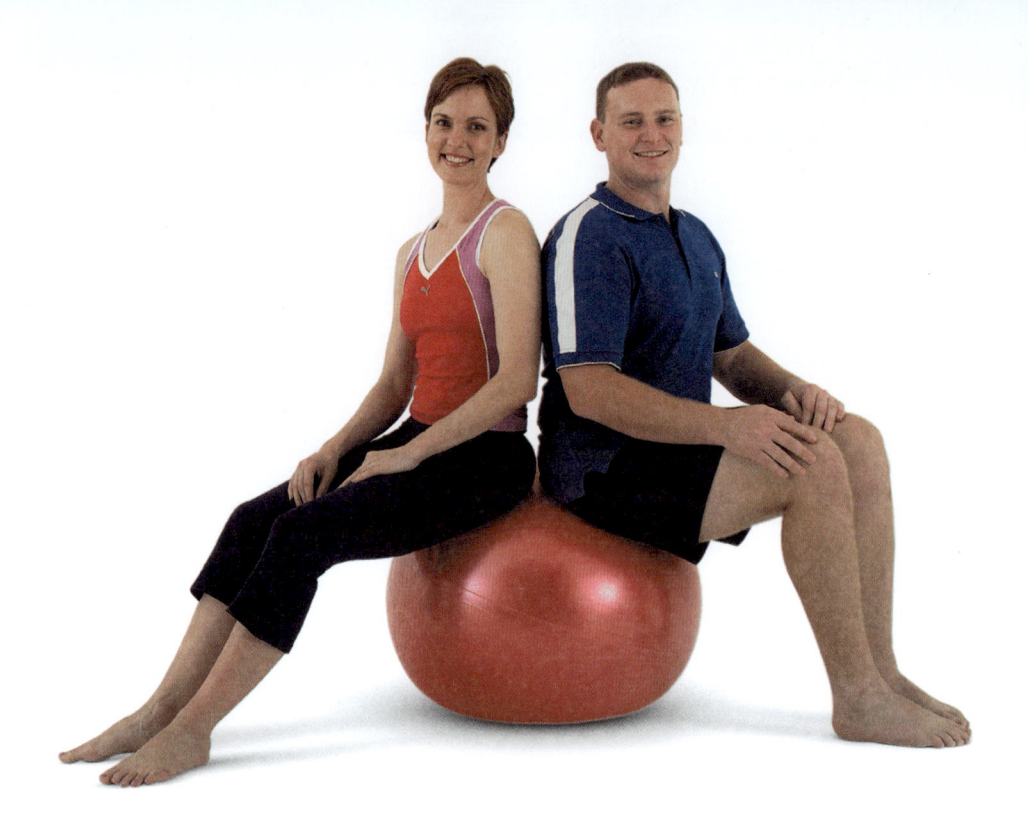

Jennifer Pohlman completed a Bachelor of Dance at the Victorian College of the Arts in Melbourne and has had over fifteen years' experience with the Pilates Method. She began Pilates training first as a dancer, as a rehabilitative measure for chronic lower-back injury. The natural progression to instructor training happened by means of an apprentice-based course oven an intensive six-month period. Following two years of teaching in a busy Pilates studio and physiotherapy centres, both in Brisbane and on the Gold Cost, Jennifer established her own business, 'Pilates InsideOut', which has been going for over a decade.

Rodney Searle has a background in various physical disciplines. Primarily a professional classical ballet dancer, he began Pilates in the late nineties, following ankle surgery while studying at the Australian Ballet School. Rodney has diversified his skills with many years of gymnastics, martial arts and various dance genres. He is a qualified instructor in the Pilates Method, having studied with Michael King (of Pilates Institute, U.K.) and instructor-trainers from Australia's Body Arts and Science and has enjoyed teaching a wide range of clients on the Gold Coast.